TABLE OF CONTENTS

Introduction Pg 1

Chapter 1	What Are Essential Oils? Pg 4
Chapter 2	Which Brands Should I Buy? Pg 8
Chapter 3	Which Essential Oils Do I Start With? Pg 12
Chapter 4	How Do I Use Essential Oils? Pg 16
Chapter 5	Inhalation Pg 19
Chapter 6	Topical Use Pg 25
Chapter 7	Ingestion and Reactions Pg 29
Chapter 8	Carrier Oils and Emulsifiers Pg 32
Chapter 9	Essential Oils While Pregnant/Breastfeeding Pg 42
Chapter 10	Essential Oils with Babies and Children Pg 59
Chapter 11	Storing, GC/MS and DIY tips Pg 71
Chapter 12	Essential Oils and their Considerations Pg 79
Chapter 13	Recipes for the Whole Family Pg 85

Final Thoughts Pg 89

Glossary Pg 91

INTRODUCTION:

Heard of essential oils? You probably have. With their popularity increasing each year, it seems that pretty much everyone knows at least something about them. You might think of a certain company, perhaps a consultant selling them, or maybe someone trying to get you to join their party or sell you some oils. That isn't what this book is about. You aren't going to be sold oils or get asked to join my team.

Despite their growing popularity, I have noticed a perplexing trend- the more people use essential oils, the less they seem to know about them. So, research is the answer… right? Well, some of the advice floating around online, on social media, and from companies that sell essential oils is not always the best. Oftentimes, this "advice" is little more than a thinly veiled effort to sell you oils or further their company. Like I said, my goal is not to make money. I want people to have the best advice to help further their aromatherapy goals, and I do not believe a hefty price tag needs to be attached.

So how does someone differentiate good from bad advice? Hello. Hi there. That is where I come in. I'm Tris, and I am a certified aromatherapist (level 2). My story begins around 2017, during my yoga teacher training, when I found some essential oils in a store and took a huge interest in them. I wanted to find more natural ways to support my health, and essential oils seemed to promise everything I was looking for. I bought those oils from the store and went on my way. I was soon told by a friend that the oils I had purchased were from a bad company, and that I needed to purchase the oils she was selling to ensure their purity. She told me that only her company's oils were pure, and that it was the only company you could trust to use, even claiming that you could use the essential oils neat (without a carrier oil) or ingest them! She then pulled out a bottle of her own oil and started dropping several drops right onto her tongue! Back then I was in awe, but now I am just scared for her and her safety if she is continuing this practice.

But okay, I'll admit it, I was intrigued at the time. I really thought that I was doing a disservice to myself by buying a bad brand. I believed what she was saying, and that she was truly trained in essential oils. I bought what she said and investigated her company. But the price tag was alarming… over $100 just to sign up with this company. And I had to sign up, I was told, or I wouldn't get the best deal. I didn't "have" to sell and was told not to worry about it and to just buy the kit. I had to purchase a certain amount every month, though (totaling between $50-$100) to remain "active" and get this amazing discount she was telling me about. All of that really put me off wanting to try them, and I slowly began to realize that her touting proudly to be an essential oil expert wasn't exactly accurate. She didn't really know what she was talking about. It wasn't until much later that I discovered the full truth about her company and how little she actually knew. It turned out that she was trained by her company. Trained to sell. But she wasn't trained in aromatherapy, how to use essential

Dedications

To my wonderful husband - I never would have made it this far in my studies and business without your undying support. You have always been there for me and supported me as I started my courses and my business.

And to my three beautiful girls - you have always shown me how to continue having fun in life and given me something to keep working towards. Thank you for all the times I used you guys as test subjects, for putting up with me constantly being on social media, and for encouraging me in all that I do.

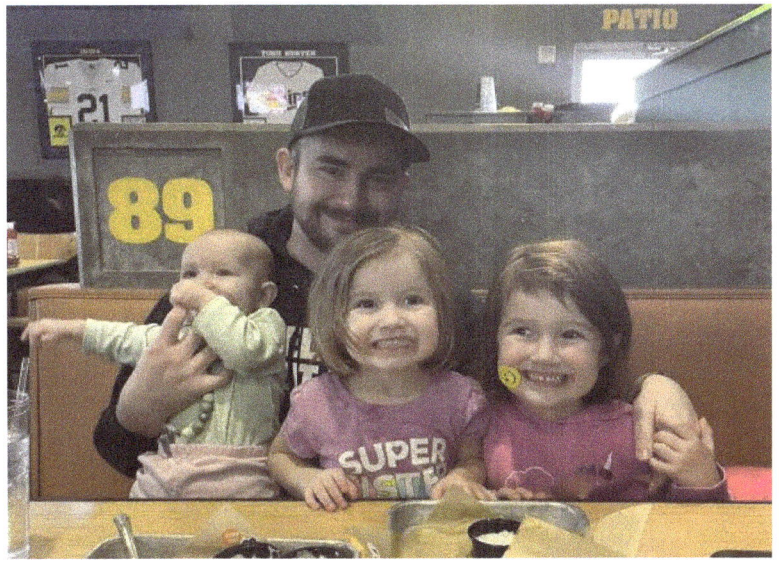

oils, or relevant safety considerations.

At the time, I was experiencing sticker shock. It was a massive price tag, accompanied by the feeling that I was being tricked into a sale. For that I am glad, because I ended up telling her I wasn't able to afford it, but that maybe I could in the future. Then I researched on my own a little bit and found other brands, with great reviews. I purchased a kit from another brand that had a much more reasonable price tag and called it a day. I used those essential oils for a while, although I will admit that I knew absolutely nothing about them. They served me well, and when I investigated the company, they seemed honest and open. When I got pregnant, I mostly stopped using oils because I didn't know which ones were actually safe and was hearing a lot of mixed things about using them during pregnancy. However, I did use them during my pregnancy on occasion and in ways that I most definitely should not have used them. If anyone wants to hear the story of when I read that peppermint essential oil stops Braxton-Hicks contractions and so dumped the undiluted oil right onto my very pregnant belly, let me know!It's certainly a cautionary tale, and something that I can now look back on and laugh at. At the time, when I was screaming that it was cold to my husband, it was less hilarious. Then there's the time I added undiluted lemongrass to my bath and ended up screaming at my husband that I was burning. You could say I'm a prime example of what not to do, but at least you can learn from me!

After my first daughter was born, I continued to use the first company I purchased from. They had a mom and baby kit (it literally said, "mama and baby", emphasis on BABY we will talk about why that word is important later on) and I was thrilled to have some baby safe essential oils to use. I trusted that they were advertising truthfully, but would later learn they were not. I joined Instagram toward the end of summer 2020, and found myself a nice little community of other essential oils users. This is where I discovered two things: 1) aromatherapy is a profession, and 2) that it was easier than I had previously thought to learn about essential oils.

Sometime after my first child, I also discovered I had scoliosis. Back pain had been a frequent companion of mine throughout my adult life, but I never received any real answers as to why it was happening. After a futile attempt to get answers from my doctor, and having steroids tossed at me, I had given up on getting any kind of help for the pain. The scoliosis diagnosis changed my life and led me to finally find things that could help me. This diagnosis prompted me to embark on a holistic journey, and that is what eventually led to my aromatherapy certification.

I began to explore options for courses and researched how I could become certified. Some online courses were more for information than certification, but they did serve to teach me that it was something I was passionate about and wanted to do. It was on this journey when I discovered that the brand of essential oils, I was using wasn't actually a good brand (remember that mama and baby kit?), and that their marketing was anything but truthful. Upon further inspection of the company, they seemed shady. There'd been several reports of adulteration in their essential oils. There was also the addition of some oils that weren't considered safe for children in their kits (remember those kits were advertised for mom and baby), and some not even safe for breastfeeding mothers. Their customer service was extremely unhelpful as well, telling me that the mom and baby kit was for ages 3+ despite being marketed towards mom and BABIES. I quickly ditched that brand and found several others that I trusted a lot more. They have stood the test of time, and even after taking a few more courses and completing two certified NAHA (National Association for Holistic Aromatherapy) certification courses, I still use and love these companies.

Getting to where I am today was a long journey, with a lot of trial and error. I am still pursuing a higher certification and working towards my clinical certification to hopefully work as a doula and utilize aromatherapy to help those going through pregnancy and childbirth. I have learned a lot, which would not have been possible without seeing the error of my past ways. I went through ups and downs, horrified myself quite a few times with some very unsafe practices, and served as my own guinea pig while learning what—and what not—to do while using essential oils.

So, if you are like me, and you have played around with essential oils but want to learn more, then this book is for you. Maybe you've used them for a while, maybe you're just getting into them. Either way, this is a great book for laying out all the ins and outs of aromatherapy, using essential oils, and knowing what is safe. I have taken the work out of getting the information you need. I am someone who believes essential oil education doesn't need to have a huge price tag, and that if you are interested in using essential oils then the safety information on them should be readily available.

CHAPTER 1: WHAT ARE ESSENTIAL OILS?

You might have been told that essential oils are called essential because we need them. I don't know how many people believe this, but I do know a lot of people joke about this. "They are called essential oils because they are essential, and we need them!" Remarks like this are usually followed by laughter.

With all things, and particularly aromatherapy, I can only assume that if someone is saying something, then they believe it to some extent. Especially if they are selling essential oils. Here's the truth. Essential oils are called essential because they are the essence of the plant. There are tiny glands, hairs, and sacs that contain this plant concentrate (the essential oil). Using methods of distillation and extraction, we collect these essential oils and bottle them. However, they weren't always so easily accessible in a bottle like they are today. Essential oils, and aromatherapy in general, have a long history. The essential oils of the past were not quite like the ones we know and use today.

A BRIEF HISTORY OF AROMATHERAPY

Aromatic herbs have been used throughout history, and their use has been recorded across different cultures and peoples. The ancient Egyptians used aromas, herbs, and oils for religious ceremonies, everyday care, and healing, and the Chinese have an extensive history of medicinal herbs. Without modern advances in the extraction of oil, the raw herbs were the go-to, and there were several ways to use them. While it would be a long while until distillation was possible, and even longer until modern distilleries came to be and essential oils were produced on a large scale, there were many ways people reaped the aromatic benefits: perfumes, incense, baths, and infused oils were common.

The Greeks used aromas for their gods as offerings, utilizing incense and perfumes. In biblical times, fresh herbs were scattered on the ground so that their aroma would be released when walked on. Many cultures used them in baths, added them to their daily routines to stay fresh/clean, and utilized the herbs for cleaning. During the black plague, herbs were stuffed into masks to help kill smells and cleanse the air.

When people say essential oils have been used for hundreds of years, it's important to realize that essential oils looked different until modern distilling methods came to be. There were major differences in aromatherapy back then. When the popularity of herbal products grew, along with widespread interest in the personal use of aromatherapy and herbs, new ways were pursued to get the most out of herbs. While aromatherapy has been used for hundreds of years, the essential oils that we know and love today are a relatively new invention. Back in the day, aromatic oils were usually expressed or extracted using fatty oils and in small quantities or steeped in a carrier oil instead of distilled as they are today. One of the most popular historical references to these healing plants (mistakenly thought of as modern-day essential oils) was the birth of Jesus and the wise men bringing him frankincense and myrrh. So, although people joke about Jesus using essential oils, this isn't quite accurate as. Again, modern essential oils as we know them just weren't a thing back then! While it's fun to joke that we are using the same oils Jesus did, it's important to know the historical truth… we are not. Jesus most likely received the entire herb/plant, or an infused oil, rather than modern distilled essential oils.

Eventually, the desire and need for herbs and herbal medicine diminished. As society advanced and modern medicines emerged, natural remedies fell into disuse. They were later picked back up again by a few who rekindled interest in them. One of the largest names that you may have heard of is Rene-Maurice Gattefosse. Maybe you have heard the now infamous story of how he just happened to have an open container of lavender essential oil on hand and, when he burned himself, he instinctively plunged his hand into the container? While it is true that he burned himself and applied lavender essential oil, then noted how it helped the healing process, the story that is shared is a bit dramatic and makes it seem like it was some miracle discovery of how great essential oils are. Instead, it is simply a tale of a calculated decision of one man studying the medicinal benefits of essential oils. With a quote from his own book, we can see the intent and the study behind such a move:

"The external application of small quantities of essences rapidly stops the spread of gangrenous sores. In my personal experience, after a laboratory explosion covered me with burning substances which I extinguished by rolling on a grassy lawn, both my hands were covered with a rapidly developing gas gangrene. Just one rinse with lavender essence stopped "the gasification of the tissue". This treatment was followed by profuse sweating, and healing began the next day (July 1910). (Gattefosse, Rene-Maurice; Aromatherapie English publication 1993)"

We can see that he was intentional about applying the lavender, and he did so in a way to study the effects. The initial burn was an accident, but everything following it was not. While the embellished story makes for a great tale and serves to generate intrigue around aromatherapy as a whole, it's just not true. It also does a disservice to the actual studies and intentions that made possible where we are today with aromatherapy.

Other leading names in aromatherapy are Dr. Jean Valnet and Marguerite Maury. Valnet was a French scientist and army physician who used essential oils to successfully treat wounded soldiers during World War Two, when antibiotics had run out. His work established the development of the modern use of essential oils as supplemental care, alongside primary healthcare. Marguerite Maury began to study how essential oils could be used to penetrate the skin during massage, which is something still being practiced today.

In today's world we have access to modern essential oils and their myriads of benefits, all backed by a long history of use and studies. But how did we go from utilizing herbs aromatically to distilling them at such a large scale? When did modern distilleries come into play and pave the way for what we know today? After the aromatherapy world had died down for a little bit, and the resurgence of herbs and oils began, a man named Ibn Sina invented a unique kind of condensing coil that made it easier and more efficient to extract essential oils from plants and herbs through steam distillation. Sina is regarded as the pioneer of aromatherapy because of this. As a result, the aromatherapy industry experienced a resurgence, and thanks to those scientists and their studies/findings it has grown to what it is today.

ESSENTIAL OILS

Essential oils are plant extracts. Through a variety of different extraction methods, the distilling process removes the essence of the plant. On a microscopic level, we can see the plants that produce these oils contain many suppositories (little pockets filled with the substance known as essential oils) within their cells. It's important to note that not every plant produces an essential oil, and some plants require more plant matter to produce each bottle of essential oil. On top of that, there are several methods that can be used to extract essential oils. Let's look at some of the most popular methods.

- **STEAM DISTILLATION:** This is the most popular way to extract essential oils. The plant matter is placed in a container and suspended over water which is then brought to a boil. As the water boils, steam passes through the plant matter and carries the essential oils to another container through a series of tubing. What's left in this container is a mix of the essential oil and water that has condensed from the steam. The water is then filtered off through a funnel in the bottom of the container, leaving only the essential oil to be bottled up. The leftover water is called a hydrosol, or floral water, and many companies also sell this, as it has many aromatherapeutic benefits as well. We will go over hydrosols more in depth later in this book (Ch. 9 &10).

- **EXPRESSION (COLD PRESSED ESSENTIAL OILS):** This method is usually reserved for citrus oils and is done by pressing the plant matter with a device with short needles, thus puncturing and forcing the oils out of the plant matter. Have you ever twisted the peel of an orange or other citrus fruit and gotten that burst of juice out of the peel? That is the essential oil of the plant, and expression is that on a larger scale. Another thing to note is that expressed essential oils tend to be phototoxic. Most citrus oils are phototoxic, and measures need to be taken to avoid a phototoxic reaction. However, not all citrus oils are phototoxic, and not all phototoxic oils are citrus oils, or even cold pressed.

- **TURBO DISTILLATION:** A faster method where plants are soaked in water and then steam is run through that. This is much like steam distillation, but with a good soaking, and is used for tougher plant materials such as barks, roots, or seeds.

- **HYDRO DIFFUSION:** This is a method of steam distillation which steams the plants from the top rather than the bottom and is considered less harsh as it covers the plant matter a little more evenly.

- **CO2 EXTRACTION:** This method uses carbon dioxide under extremely high pressure to extract essential oil. The plant matter is enclosed in a stainless-steel tank which is then filled with CO2 and pressurized. The CO2 then acts as solvent and extracts the oils as it turns to liquid. It then returns to a gas state (as the pressure is lessened) and leaves behind no residue. There is a higher yield of oil with this method, and that oil has a crisper smell and is a little more potent.

So, now we know what essential oils are, we know how they came to be what they are today, and how they are extracted and collected. There is certainly more that we could cover, but for this book we are only going to cover the basics necessary to begin building that foundation to using essential oils safely. Unless you are becoming a certified aromatherapist, you don't need every single minute detail of the essential oil process.

CHAPTER 2: WHICH BRANDS SHOULD I BUY?

What brand should I buy? This is one of the biggest questions asked in aromatherapy, and within it are all kinds of other questions, like, what brand is worth the money, the purest, the best quality? There honestly isn't a one size fits all answer to these, and while there are ways to determine if an essential oil is of good quality or not, the brand that you buy is entirely up to you and your preferences. As long as you are sure of its quality, then there really isn't a singular brand that is "the best."

But people still like to claim otherwise. There has been much debate on this topic, and many companies will make claims on the purity of their essential oils and market theirs to be the best or the "only" pure brand. This is simply a sales tactic, and oftentimes the marketing or language that they use to sell their products aren't legitimate. The FDA doesn't control, regulate, or approve of any essential oils at this given time. So, while that means essential oils are freely sold, there is no regulation when it comes to how they are marketed. You might have heard that some essential oil brands are "FDA approved" and this is just not the case. Since the FDA doesn't regulate essential oils, they also don't approve or disapprove them! Instead, there are some basic guidelines that need to be followed if the essential oils fall under certain categories, such as supplements. This just means that the FDA can't really do anything if the company follows some very basic labeling guidelines. The best that can be said about some essential oil brands is that they are FDA compliant. So, for example, if a company has a product that would be considered a dietary supplement, they must have that product separately labeled as a supplement. Even if they are the exact same product as one that is not a supplement. You aren't allowed to market essential oils as a supplement without the correct labeling. Instead, a company must create a special supplement line that clarifies that it is for ingestion only and follows labeling laws. Most companies simply state on the bottle they are not for ingestion. Many people believe this means the oils aren't pure, but this isn't the case. They are simply following labeling laws. This also protects companies in the eventuality that if someone were to ingest their essential oils and try to sue them for any harmful effects, they would be unable to if the bottle was clearly labeled "not for ingestion".

This has led to a lot of confusion in the sale of essential oils, and even confusion on which oils are pure. Some oils are still regarded as purer or of a higher quality because companies market them as supplements, market them as purer options, or they use trademarked wording to sell their essential oils. Unfortunately, like I said before, this doesn't really mean anything. Remember, there is no regulatory body that determines if what they are selling is actually the best quality. Luckily, there are many ways to tell if an essential oil is from a good brand. Personal preference comes into play here as well.

So, how can we tell if an essential oil is the real deal? There are a few things to look for; some green flags, if you will. If an oil is lacking this information, either on the bottle or on the website, I personally wouldn't purchase it. That doesn't mean if some of this information is missing it is an automatic red flag, this is just what I look for when purchasing. This is the golden standard for essential oils. There are still some things that, personally, I wouldn't sacrifice when looking for essential oils. However, there can be companies that don't meet my criteria and still produce great oils. If a company is missing this information, simply reach out to them and ask. If they can provide you the answers you are looking for then they are most likely legitimate.

HOW TO TELL IF AN ESSENTIAL OIL IS PURE, OR OF GOOD QUALITY:

- Origin: Most essential oil companies will list the origin of the plant used for their essential oil. This one isn't quite as important when deciding if it's a company you would like to use, however I do find it to be helpful. It can help pinpoint where/how they source, and even the therapeutic qualities of the essential oil in the bottle. Sometimes the exact same essential oil can differ slightly from batch to batch or company to company because of when and where it was harvested. There is a range of normal for which components make up each specific essential oil, the origin of the plant can give insight on if the constituents (the chemical make-up of the oil) are in that normal range. Sometimes essential oils can only be found in certain areas as well, so this can help ensure that the company is being open/honest and not just making things up. There are also essential oils that are endangered or over-harvested and knowing this information can help us ensure the company is operating sustainably and honestly.

- GC/MS reports: This is the big one for me. Do I thoroughly read every single one? Honestly, no. Oftentimes I just ask if they have them, and then look over them briefly but I don't read them on every oil I purchase. If they openly admit that they have them and don't feel the need to hide, to me that means that they are an open and honest company. Just knowing that they are easily accessible can be enough for me. Some companies will offer them, but only if you purchase first. Some companies won't offer them at all. Some companies don't have them but are still open if you ask them about it and will tell you anything you want to know regardless. If a company can't give you basic information (at the very least) on the quality and contents of their essential oil, I wouldn't trust them. I fully believe that reports should be freely available 100% of the time, even before purchase. It is a disservice to the consumer to not have full transparency on what they are purchasing. It is up to you to decide if you are comfortable with companies withholding GC/MS reports until you purchase, although I personally do not like this.

- Distillation: On the website, their method of distillation should be listed. If the company doesn't distill themselves, then there should be links to the information about where they source their essential oils. This is mostly just nice to know, but also because some essential oils can be distilled in more than one way and depending on how it was distilled this can change the essential oil slightly. Some essential oils are phototoxic (they react in sunlight) when distilled in certain ways, some are more expensive with certain distillation methods, etc. It's nice to know about the oil you are purchasing and helps ensure safety.

- Latin names/botanical names: You will find that most essential oils have Latin names on the bottle (or at the very least on the website, but preferably on the bottle). This is one of those things that I do not overlook. If it doesn't have the Latin name, don't purchase it. Even if the oil is pure or of good quality, we do not know its Latin name and therefore will not always know how to appropriately use it. Sometimes, there are several different types under a single species, and they sometimes have different considerations for using them. Like lavender, for example - there are several variations such as English lavender, Spanish lavender, Spike lavender, and lavandin (which is a lavender hybrid). If the bottle just says lavender, I wouldn't know if I was using a lavender or a lavender hybrid. It's important to know which plant we are using. Why? Well, if it's lavandin we need to know because it can be an anticoagulant. If it's Spanish lavender, that can be a convulsant. These are very different effects, so it's important to know exactly what we are using to ensure our safety!
- Safety: There absolutely should be safety information on the essential oil that you are using. They should have comprehensive safety information on their website, but at least basic safety on the bottle is a must. Is this kid safe? Pregnancy safe? Can it be used while breastfeeding? Is it animal safe? Is this essential oil contraindicated for those with any medical conditions, who take any medicines, or use any other products? These are things that consumers must know, and it is expected that companies will share. Below I share an example of a good essential oil bottle with all the information needed on the bottle.

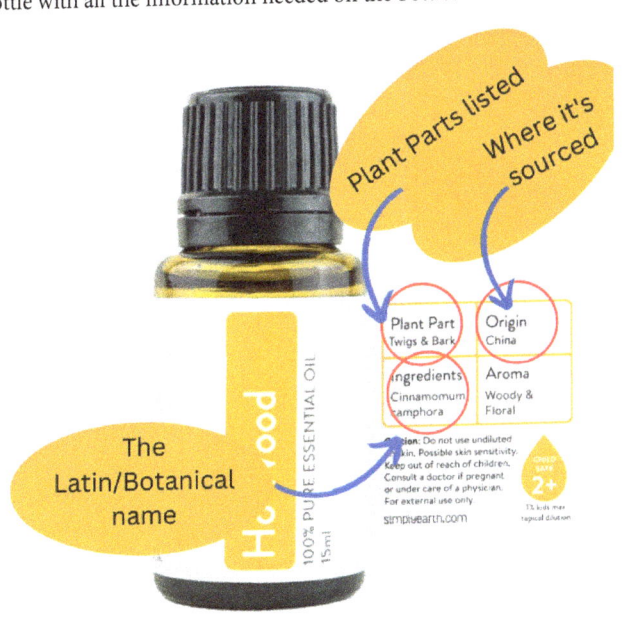

These are my top ways to determine a good essential oil company. There will be a lot of backlash surrounding certain companies, especially in an online setting. People have opinions and they love to share them. People also love to harp on others for not sharing the same opinion. Having a preference is fine, but problems arise when companies try to battle for the best spot and try to make it seem like they are the only good company or even try to spread lies about other companies. Objectively, it's easy to look at a company and determine if it's one you want to use. For these reasons, I won't be sharing my favorite companies. I am open about them on my website and social media, but for the purposes of this book I shall remain brandless. Use the tools in this book to find the best company for you, and in the process remain aware that the opinions of others doesn't paint the full picture of essential oil companies, or even essential oils as a whole.

You will also find that aromatherapists have opinions on which brand is best, and that some just don't care which brand you use. Don't let their opinions sway you. While there is nothing wrong with using a company because someone you trust prefers a that company, it is important not to demonize other companies just because it gets hate from someone else. Alongside that, we also shouldn't idolize a company just because it gets a lot of favor. Any company has the potential to be good or bad, and it's important to know how to look for quality in a company in these cases. For the most part, there are several brands and companies that are great, and in the end, it really boils down to preference.

CHAPTER 3: WHICH ESSENTIAL OILS DO I START WITH?

Which oils should I get? This is my second most-asked question. Which really, if we unpack that, it is also asking a few other questions as well: What are the best essential oils to start with? How many do I need? What are some good oils to keep on hand? With so many companies selling and pushing their oils, it can be super overwhelming to know which ones to start with, which ones you might need, and which are best not bought at all. As stated in previous chapters, essential oils are not regulated, which is great for a free market, but not so great when companies start selling things that probably shouldn't be available to the public in such large quantities. So, what essential oils should you get, as someone just starting out?

I always recommend a top five essential oil list to people. These are five staple essential oils to have on hand that will work for most things people are looking to use essential oils for. One of the biggest misconceptions in the aromatherapy/essential oil world is that you need a lot of different ones. This is a common myth that is propagated by essential oil companies, mostly to get people to buy more products. Alongside some questionable advice on how to use oils, these companies encourage us to collect oils rather than treat them as a medicinal tool or therapeutic modality. This isn't to say essential oils can entirely replace medicine, just that they should be treated as such and used sparingly. We don't go to a drugstore and clean out every type of medicine they offer, and we don't collect each brand or type. Likewise, we certainly don't need to stockpile bottle after bottle of every single kind of essential oil available for purchase!

Another reason to avoid stockpiling is that oils have a shelf life, and that is something I will discuss in a later chapter (Ch. 11). It doesn't make sense to have hundreds of different oils, or multiple bottles of the same oil "just in case". They would more than likely reach the end of their shelf life before you ever get to them. They are a finite resource, and many of them are hard to find because of over-harvesting. If you don't need it, don't get it. Buying something just to have it, to display a pretty bottle, or to add to a collection is detrimental to the environment and plant life. On top of that, in order to use up so many bottles of essential oil in a timely manner a person would have to overuse them to such an extreme that they would be at risk of experiencing adverse reactions. So, as an aromatherapist, here are the top 5 essential oils I recommend for beginners.

MY TOP FIVE ESSENTIAL OILS:

1.) Tea tree (Melaleuca alternifolia): Tea Tree is a super useful oil; great for dandruff, skin issues, head lice, cold/flu season, and even fungal infections. It's also a good cleaning oil, and great for diffusing to clean up the air a little bit. It has so many uses that I could write an entire chapter on this oil alone. This is one of the top oils that I recommend to people, and it's one of the few that I actually use up relatively quickly. It isn't my favorite scent, but it is incredibly useful.

2.) Roman chamomile (Anthemis nobilis): My love of chamomile knows no bounds, and it's one of my go-to oils for first aid. It helps sore muscles, is good for bruises, is a skin soothing/healing oil, and is a wonderfully calming oil which makes it amazing for bedtime. I find I like chamomile so much more than lavender essential oil. It's also great for kids, since some children do not respond well to lavender oil. Children with ADHD (or other neuro-divergence) might become hyper or agitated with lavender essential oil.

3.) Lemon (Citrus x limon): I had to have a citrus oil in the mix. It's great for cleaning, and citrus oils also tend to be a mood lifter and can brighten up the day. I love diffusing lemon while cleaning for a fresh scent, and it's a good boost for cleaning products if you make your own. I would mix lemon with tea tree in some castile soap for a great hand soap option as well. While lemon isn't an oil I turn to super often, it is one I would still miss if I didn't always have it on hand.

4.) Rosemary (Rosmarinus officinalis): Rosemary has helped me many times with my back pain, specifically nerve pain. It's great for the muscles, nerves, stimulating hair growth, memory, and digestion. This would be a great one to use for a massage when blended with some carrier oil. It is often overlooked, but I think it has a lot of potential. However, this is the only one on this list that isn't traditionally kid safe, so be wary of that. Pay close attention to the chemical makeup of the rosemary that you choose. Some companies have a rosemary option that is a cineole 1,8 chemotype (this just refers to which chemical constituent is most prominent in the essential oil) and this is definitely not kid safe. If you're wanting a similar, kid safe option, spearmint would be great for sore muscles/pain, memory/alertness, and digestion as well. There are also other chemotypes of rosemary that are much safer (such as the camphor chemotype), although they are a little harder to find.

5.) Ho wood (Cinnamomum camphor): My favorite oil in the calming department is ho wood, and it is our go-to for bedtime. It comes from the cinnamon family, and you can definitely tell. It has a rich, herby/woody scent that I can only describe as being the same kind of heaviness you get when you smell or taste black licorice. But don't fear, it's nothing like licorice! This oil is so calming and so wonderful, making it perfect for bedtime or sore muscles rubs. It's a much better oil than lavender and way more effective in the calming department in my opinion. I highly recommend this for a good bedtime oil, and the best part is that it's absolutely kid safe. This oil is also a fantastic replacement for the endangered rosewood essential oil.

    This list can certainly be played around with as well. It includes ones that I enjoy, and also offers a variety of choices. You could replace ho wood with lavender if you still want a sleepy time essential oil that is a little more versatile. It is good to note that lavender, while providing notable sleep inducing and calming effects, does not always have these effects on everyone. Another thing to keep in mind is that this list is pretty safe, with all oils (apart from rosemary) being safe for all ages and having little to no contraindications, even in the case of those who are pregnant/breastfeed ing (not on a clinical level) to whom they pose little to no risk. I will detail more on how to use these essential oils and their safety in later chapters (Ch. 9, 10, & 12). If you are looking for a good staple set of oils that is generally regarded as safe, this list is it. They cover a multitude of issues, from physical to emotional, and are generally a great starting point for every person and family. Most starter packs on an essential oil company's site will contain these oils or similar, plus some blends, and are also a good choice for getting started. If you don't want to buy single oils, starter kits are usually a great deal and make it easy to get started with essential oils.

SAFETY CONSIDERATIONS:

- Tea tree: Topical max is 15%, safe during pregnancy (not clinically studied) and breastfeeding, safe for all ages, and safe for dogs. Shelf life is 2 years.
- Spearmint (as an alternative to rosemary): Topical max is 1.7%, safe during pregnancy (not clinically studied) and breastfeeding, safe for all ages, and safe for dogs. Shelf life is 4 years.
- Rosemary 1,8 cineole: No topical max but always dilute, safe during pregnancy (not clinically studied) and breastfeeding, safe for ages 10+, and safe for dogs. Shelf life is 3 years.
- Rosemary ct camphor: Topical max 16.5%, safe during pregnancy (not clinically studied) and breastfeeding, safe for all ages, and safe for dogs. Shelf life 3 years
- Roman chamomile: No topical max but always dilute, safe during pregnancy (not clinically studied) and breastfeeding, safe for all ages, and safe for dogs. Shelf life is 7 years.
- Lemon: Topical max is 2%, safe during pregnancy (clinically studied) and breastfeeding, safe for all ages, and safe for dogs. Lemon is a phototoxic oil, meaning it will cause a reaction on the skin when exposed to UV rays. Apply 12 hours before going into the sun, or on areas not exposed to UV rays. Follow the topical max to avoid a reaction. Shelf life is 2 years.
- Ho wood: No topical max but always dilute before applying to the skin. Safe during pregnancy (not clinically studied) and breastfeeding, safe for all ages. Avoid using this around your pets. Shelf life is 3 years.

I will go over the safe use of essential oils while diffusing and when applying topically in later chapters (Ch. 5,6, & 7). This is just the general safety profile for each oil I mentioned, and it is important to note the chemotypes of rosemary, as they are for different purposes, although generally they will do the same things. Some chemotypes are just better for certain conditions, such as cineole being best for respiratory and camphor for muscular/nerve pains. Camphor is safe for kids, but cineole is not. If you want to stock all kid safe essential oils, then substitute the rosemary essential oil for Spearmint (as mentioned above).

I would also like to note that pet safe essential oils require proper care and use. This is not something that I will be covering in this book, as I am not trained in that area. If it is listed as pet safe, then please take that to mean that it is safe to diffuse around pets so long as the room gets a lot of airflow, and the pet is allowed to leave. Please note that cats lack the enzyme that processes essential oils, so there are no essential oils that are safe for cats, and even some they need to avoid altogether. As mentioned, this is not something I am trained in, and it is best to contact your vet for clarification and avoid diffusing around cats/rodents/fish/small mammals.

CHAPTER 4: HOW DO I USE ESSENTIAL OILS?

We have covered what essential oils are, how to choose a brand, and what essential oils to have on hand. But how can we use these oils? If you have never really done anything with essential oils, this question can seem intimidating. With rampant misinformation floating around out there, it can also be hard to know what is actually safe and what is just marketing propaganda. I will only be covering American aromatherpay usage in these chapters, that is what I am trained in.

METHODS OF USE

Aromatically: Aromatic covers all uses where you would inhale the essential oils - diffusers, personal inhalers, steaming, etc. There are so many ways, and these will be covered in their own chapter (Ch. 5).

Topically: Topical use means all the ways in which you use oils by applying to skin to treat physical pains, etc. More options and in-depth descriptions of how to utilize essential oils topically in later chapters (Ch. 6).

Internally: Internal use of essential oils covers ingestion, including doing so vaginally, with suppositories, etc. and will not be detailed in this book. You shouldn't use essential oils internally without the help and guidance of a certified clinical aromatherapist. It is not recommended to use essential oils in this manner (in American aromatherapy), or to utilize essential oils internally for any length of time/daily use. There will be a chapter on ingestion, but it will be about safety and caution on casual and daily ingestion (Ch. 7).

There are many different ways to apply these methods, and they will be briefly covered in this chapter. I will also note some of my favorite methods and which are best for addressing certain issues.

AROMATICALLY

There are a few different ways to go about inhaling essential oils, the most popular being with a diffuser. There are also personal inhalers, passive diffusers, and diffuser jewelry - these methods being the most well-known. Diffusing is when you add essential oils to a machine (or object) that holds water and then steams the essential oils out. This is one of the best and most efficient methods of inhalation. There are several different types of diffusers such as evaporative, ultrasonic, nebulizers, reed diffusers, passive diffusers, personal inhalers, and diffuser jewelry. Personal inhalers are a great way to enjoy the benefits of essential oils on the go. Diffuser jewelry can also do that; however, it doesn't last as long and could potentially disturb other people. You can also do a steaming session with essential oils, either by adding some oils to your shower or by using the bowl and towel method with hot water to steam.

Passive diffusers are also a great method, especially for small spaces. All of these options are great ways to utilize essential oils aromatically, and I will go over these methods in greater detail in the appropriate chapter (Ch. 5).

TOPICAL

Topical use is just that - using essential oils topically (on skin). You can use all kinds of carriers, from lotions to oils (olive, coconut, grapeseed, almond, etc.), and you can get as creative as you like with this. You could choose something as simple as a carrier oil, use a basic lotion base, or even make your own base like body butter. This can really be as complicated or simple as you want. There are so many different ways to utilize essential oils topically, and they will be covered in a subsequent chapter (Ch. 6).

Again, for the sake of safety, I will not talk about ingestion. While there are ways to ingest oils safely, I am not trained in these methods. Even when I finish my clinicals and become trained/certified to do so, I wouldn't recommend someone ingest essential oils by simply following the guidance of a book because there can be some negative outcomes that really require in person guidance. As I mentioned before, if you want to use essential oils internally, then contact someone appropriately trained. And make sure that person is a clinical aromatherapist, as they are trained in the medical aspects of aromatherapy and have the appropriate knowledge. Ingestion is never something that should be done casually or daily. It has its time and place, certainly, but it needs to be done in a safe manner. Most of the information that people share on ingesting essential oils comes from large companies trying to sell their oils and can end up causing some serious side effects. People rarely stop to consider the consequences of ingesting something as potent as an essential oil in a careless manner.

With so many ways to utilize essential oils, it can be hard to know what the right method is. An easy way I like to remember what methods work best for what issue is this: emotional or respiratory issues are best addressed through inhalation, and physical ailments and germ defense mean topical use. This isn't a hard and fast rule. For example, sometimes for respiratory issues I find a nice balm works best and that for an emotional issue, adding essential oils to the bath can help (the bath can count as topical and aromatic use). My favorite method of use for myself is topical. As someone who experiences a lot of pain, the topical method works wonders for me. However, I prefer using essential oils aromatically for my kids. Whatever method you find you love, be sure to engage in it safely.

For some extra information, I will add a flow chart on the different herbal products and how to utilize them to end this chapter. It is important to note which herbal products exist and how/when we can use them. I find this chart helpful, especially when deciding when to use essential oils. This also gives us an idea of how potent essential oils are compared to other herbal products. Use this chart when determining if you need to use essential oils.

Herbal Chart
Which herbal item is strongest

1.) ESSENTIAL OIL
Strongest, concentrated plant matter. One drop is equal to multiple doses of the plant

2.) HERBAL TINCTURE
Second strongest, herbal extract. Alcohol extracts the plant properties and provides and adequate dose. Ideal for internal use.

3.) HERBAL INFUSED OIL
Third strongest, oil extracts the herbal properties although not as good as alcohol. Good for topical or internal use.

4.) HYDROSOL
Weaker, this is the leftover plant matter (water) from extracting essential oils. Contains many benefits of the oils and plants but at a much lighter dose. Ideal for babies/children and pets.

5.) TEA
Weakest, provides a small extraction of the herb through hot water. Great choice for internal use. Ideal for babies/children and pets.

CHAPTER 5: INHALATION

We already know some of the main ways that we can utilize inhalation - diffusers, personal inhalers, passive diffusers, diffuser jewelry, etc. But how exactly do we use each of those? What is too much when it comes to diffusing? How much should you put on diffuser jewelry? This can all seem so intimidating if you don't know where to start, and sometimes companies don't always share the best advice. But once you get the hang of using essential oils aromatically it can be really easy, and it's one of my favorite ways to utilize them.

Inhalation is generally best when targeting emotional or respiratory issues. While this isn't an official rule, if you want the best results, using your oils aromatically will absolutely be best since there really isn't anything physical to address. Why? Well, with emotional issues, smelling works the best because of our olfactory system. Our sense of smell is heavily connected to our brains via the olfactory system. Smells alone can have a powerful effect on the mind, and certain essential oils have properties that help with certain things. For example, lemon essential oil has calming properties, so while it can be applied topically, inhaling can work wonders for calming down. In fact, lemon is better used aromatically anyways, due to its phototoxic properties. The particles from the essential oil will travel through the respiratory system, reach the olfactory system, and then spread their calming properties to the rest of the brain. The olfactory system is also why smells or aromas have such a strong correlation with memories and can bring back old memories so vividly. Since the olfactory system is connected to your entire brain, smells can bring out certain memories and feelings. This helps to explain why we have favorite smells and even dislike certain smells if it reminds us of something unpleasant.

This is all in simple terms, to make this as easy to understand as possible. I could go into a lot more detail and give you the entire workings of the brain system, but quite honestly, we don't need to go over that to understand that smells can be converted in the mind. On top of that, the science is still somewhat of a mystery when it comes to explaining how a smell ends up in the memory and feeling portions of our minds. In the absolute simplest terms, smells travel up the nose, are processed by the olfactory bulb, and are then processed by our brain. Essential oils that contain certain properties are extremely helpful when smelling, especially with issues like emotional or respiratory ailments. So then, how can we utilize the different methods of inhalation?

DIFFUSING

Sadly, there is a lot of misinformation when it comes to essential oils, and the topic of diffusing is probably the greatest minefield! You have probably bought a diffuser and noticed that it has a 1-, 2-, or 3-hour function. Perhaps it just runs until it's empty and has no other options besides on/off. You also might have noticed that if you leave the diffuser running for as long as most diffusers can go, it might be over whelming, maybe you get a headache, or maybe you just get sick of the scent after a while. The smell also doesn't dissipate right away after stopping the diffuser, especially if you've been letting it run for hours. So, how can we avoid reactions like this? Yes, they are reactions. We want to use oils in a safe way to avoid these reactions. There are also several types of diffusers, the most popular being ultrasonic diffusers. For simplicity, I will be covering ultrasonic diffusers because they are the most readily available and most easily accessible diffusers.

Pick a diffuser that has options that benefit you: A lot of diffusers really lack in the settings department, but there are a few that have on/off auto options and limit their runtime. You want to look for one that has increments of time less than 1 hour. It's not ideal to let the diffuser run for a full hour, but this is much better than having a diffuser that never shuts off. My favorite diffuser is the portable one from Plant Therapy, as it has the best options. This diffuser cycles through for 30 minutes on then 30 minutes off, with other options alternating between on/off in varying time frames but never exceeding 30 consecutive minutes. It also doesn't need to be plugged in, and is rechargeable, so this makes it an ideal option if you can't have something plugged in where you intend to use it.

Less is more: Oftentimes it is recommended to put upwards of 10 drops into a diffuser. Depending on your diffuser size, this could seriously overpower a room very quickly! An average recommendation is 3-5 drops per 100 ml, so you will want to know your diffuser's capacity, and base it off that. Smaller diffusers only need 1-3 drops. In my travel diffuser, 1 drop is more than enough. I usually stick with 3-5 in my diffusers, because I find more than that to just be too much. If you struggle with getting the correct number of drops with individual oils, consider buying or making blends. This approach will allow you to diffuse multiple oils without having to add too many drops. Instead of having to add 3-5 drops of each oil, you can combine them into a blend and add 3-5 drops of that blend.

Consider the time you spend diffusing. Is it more than 30 minutes? You can get the best results doing 30 minutes or less. You only need about 15 minutes to get therapeutic benefits. If you want to run your diffuser for longer, consider adding fewer drops. Remember to shut the diffuser off if you feel any reactions, are getting sick of the scent, or you notice any brain fogginess associated with diffusing.

Consider the ages of the people you want to diffuse around: For older and younger people, diffuse less, with less drops, and for lower amounts of time. You can diffuse starting from around 3 months old (although you don't really need to use essential oils with babies, and I will be covering child safe aromatherapy later in chapter 10), but I don't recommend just starting off immediately with a full 30 minutes of diffusing time. Start with 1 or 2 drops in a diffuser, of a single oil. Run for 5 minutes at first. Work your way up to 15 minutes, and always watch for reactions. For older people and children, use less drops and run for 15 minutes max. We don't want to overwhelm anyone. We want to take care and exercise caution when diffusing, and using oils in general, around children and the elderly. I will talk about this more in later chapters (Ch. 6 & 10).

Consider what is being put into the diffuser. Carrier oils do not belong in diffusers. Essential oils, absolutes, and extracts only. Some companies use extracts in their blends; these are safe to diffuse. Carrier oils are thicker and will clog a diffuser. Many companies dilute their blends but are not open about the substance used to dilute (aka they used a carrier oil to cut the essential oil) so it's important to watch for this. They will (usually) list the carrier oil in the ingredients even if they don't say that it's a diluted oil and sadly these oils are not for diffusing in a water diffuser as they will eventually clog your machine. Some companies will never disclose if an oil is diluted or not so make sure the company you purchase from is legitimate and that they have GC/MS reports.

Lastly, consider the oils you are using: Many oils are safe for everyone, but many are not. Know what is safe, and keep in mind that just because it is safe doesn't mean you won't have reactions. Consider that some oils might not be good to diffuse in your home. Some oils, like cinnamon, are more prone to cause reactions, so just be cautious of what you are diffusing and keep in mind that allergic reactions can and do occur. We will discuss essential oils and relevant safety considerations in a later chapter (Ch.12).

PERSONAL INHALERS

Personal inhalers are one of my absolute favorite ways to enjoy the aromatic benefits of essential oils. They are small, portable, easy to use, and allow you to utilize essential oils in a way that will not disturb those around you or overwhelm you.

With an inhaler, there are two options: a plastic disposable inhaler and a metal reusable one. Both of these options rely on a cotton wick and can be found at several retailers including Amazon, essential oil shops, and essential oil supply shops. To use an inhaler, take the cotton wick and place in a glass container to fill. Drop the oils you desire onto the wick in the container, use some tweezers to help soak up all the oils, and then place the wick into the inhaler and seal it off. To use the inhaler, simply remove the cap, hold it under your nose, and inhale deeply for several seconds. Do this 1-3 times, repeating as needed throughout the day.

When filling a personal inhaler, it's important to note who the inhaler is for and how many drops you will want to use for that person. For the average adult, I would do 15 drops. I don't recommend the use of an inhaler by anyone under the age of 6, simply because it is still something with essential oils and young children might put it in their mouth. If you choose to use one with a child over that age, use 5-10 drops instead. For someone older (over the age of 60), also use 5-10 drops. As people age, they can become more sensitive to essential oils, just like children are more sensitive to essential oils. The essential oil also might be more easily absorbed by the body in a person who is younger/older, so it's incredibly important to consider the relation between dosage and age.

DIFFUSER JEWELRY

Diffuser jewelry is a great way to take essential oils on the go, and also be cute/trendy. It's a nice way to play around with aromatic use and add to your style. There are diffuser bracelets, necklaces, and even earrings. All of these are great ways to use essential oils aromatically. When used properly, they can also be a safe way to take essential oils on the go.

To use diffuser jewelry, simply add 1-2 drops onto the diffuser part of the jewelry item. Which part that is can vary, but it will usually be a lava bead (a porous bead), a wood bead, or some kind of macramé. You want to take care not to drop essential oils onto your skin, as all essential oils that are used topically should be diluted, so I recommend applying the oil and then putting the jewelry on. Alternatively, you can apply the essential oil with a roller bottle, but most rollers tend to be diluted already and might weaken the smell on the jewelry. Another thing that was popular for a while in the aromatherapy world was using one's hair to diffuse, either by dropping some oil onto the ends of the hair or dropping oil directly onto the scalp. I do not recommend this method, as it can be dangerous and cause reactions to the scalp. It can also be overwhelming. Consider how you can take jewelry off quickly… but you cannot just remove your hair (unless you cut it) and you can quickly become annoyed by a scent or just want to take a break. It is best to leave wearable diffusing to actual jewelry.

PASSIVE DIFFUSION

Passive diffusion might just be the easiest form of diffusing, and methods of doing so are varied. Diffuser jewelry is actually a form of passive diffusion. You can use stones or macramé items; some people even use wood. You can buy a passive diffuser or make your own. Most essential oil retailers will offer one. Usually, passive diffusers are some kind of clay/plaster or stone that absorbs the essential oil and then allows the smell to permeate the room. Passive diffusion is another one of my favorite methods because it can be great for small spaces and not be so overwhelming.

To use a passive diffuser, drop a few drops onto the stone, macramé, or wood part of the diffuser and enjoy - that's it! It allows the aroma of your essential oil to gradually waft around the room so you can enjoy a passive diffusion experience. Add fewer drops for a more subtle smell; add a few more drops for a stronger smell. Please note that you cannot turn this diffuser off, so if you add too many drops it might become overwhelming.
For a typical passive diffuser, I recommend 2-5 drops. More than that will be far too overpowering.

STEAMS

Steam treatments are another method of inhalation. There are a few different ways we can utilize a steam treatment, as well, such as the bowl steam method or the shower steam method, or some humidifiers allow you to add essential oils.

To use the bowl method, heat some water to just before its boiling point. You want it hot enough to not cool down quickly, but not so hot that you could burn yourself or waste essential oils, as too much heat can kill the scent of essential oils. Add the water to a large bowl, filled about halfway. Then add your essential oils of choice (I recommend 2-5 drops), lean over the bowl, and take a towel to cover the back of your head, keeping the steam from escaping. Breathe deeply for 10-20 minutes. Be wary of the possibility of essential oils irritating the eyes. It's best to use only a few drops and keep your eyes closed while doing a steam treatment.

To do a shower steam, add up to 5 drops of essential oils to your shower. You can either take a shower as normal, or just sit in the bathroom letting the shower run on hot and steam the essential oils into the air. If you choose to shower as normal, make sure not to drop the essential oils where you will be stepping! You should also then only add 1-3 drops. If you aren't taking a shower, and are simply allowing the shower to steam, you can add a few more drops (up to 5). Let the shower and oils steam for 10-20 minutes, or until the smell dissipates.

To use essential oils with a humidifier, see the instructions for your machine. Each one is different, and you need to follow the manufacturer's recommendations regarding using essential oils with them. Do not add essential oils to a humidifier unless it says you can. Only add these to the water base if directed to do so. Usually, there is a little tray where the steam comes out to put medicines or essential oils.

The steam methods are best for congestion and respiratory issues. The heat from the steam will help to loosen congestion/build up and if you choose essential oils that work with respiratory issues this can also help to clear things up and work as an expectorant to clear any gunk from your airways.

CROSSOVER METHODS

Some methods have dual purposes, which can be considered different methods. For example, a balm would be considered topical use, but it can also be utilized for inhalation. If you make a balm for congestion to use topically, one of the main purposes would also be inhaling the essential oils. Much like Vicks Vapor Rub, rubbing a balm for congestion on your chest can also be another method in which someone could utilize inhalation. Sometimes inhalation can contribute to pain relief, even though the general rule of thumb is to use topical treatments for pain relief. Clinical aromatherapy often focuses on aromatic use to help relieve pain, for example.

You might see aromatherapists knocking methods like this, because for some it doesn't make sense to use something topically when inhalation would be the best. Personally, I don't see an issue with this. Sometimes a balm can be a little easier to use, especially with children. You can also add herbs to your balm that would be great for topical use. Instead of running a diffuser, especially at nighttime, you can utilize an herbal balm. As long as topical dilutions are followed, and you are using essential oils appropriately, it really doesn't matter if you want to use a balm for inhalation. Do what works for you, and don't let other people's overbearing opinions bring you down! If you are being safe, that is all that matters. I once had another aromatherapist tell me that an herbal balm I had made was ineffective for congestion. That same herbal balm went on to help clear rounds of congestion during our typical winter sniffles. Wichever method you decide to use for inhalation, make sure you are being safe and using the method in the most effective and accessible way for you.

CHAPTER SIX: TOPICAL USE

Topical use means any way you use essential oils on your skin or hair. Always dilute when using topically, and always follow dilution rates and topical maxes. I have included a dilution chart and a topical max chart for reference. You can also download this chart for free on my website www.holisticaryaromatherapy.com so make sure to grab one to print out for home use.

Dilution chart

1%
10ml/2tsp= 3 drops
15ml/3tsp= 4 drops
30ml/6tsp/1oz= 9 drops

2%
10ml/2tsp= 6 drops
15ml/3tsp= 8 drops
30ml/6tsp/1oz= 18 drops

3%
10ml/2tsp= 9 drops
15ml/3tsp= 12 drops
30ml/6tsp/1oz= 27 drops

5%
10ml/2tsp= 15 drops
15ml/3tsp= 20 drops
30ml/6tsp/1oz= 45 drops

10%
10ml/2tsp= 30 drops
15ml/3tsp= 40 drops
30ml/6tsp/1oz= 90 drops

Having a dilution chart to refer to is helpful (just add the specified number of drops of oil to the amount of carrier oil according to the chart) because dilution can be tricky, especially with so many recipes online with absurd dilutions! Popular advice is that essential oils are natural, and so don't need to be diluted; they can be used at high dilutions, and they won't cause any adverse reactions. This just isn't the case. Essential oils do need to be diluted. Oils can be diluted by mixing them with an appropriate carrier oil, and we will go over carrier oils and their benefits in a later chapter (Ch. 8).

1%: Daily use, and for use with kids 2+. It is also the recommended dilution for facial applications, during pregnancy, for the elderly (60+), deodorants, and daily lotions. For kids 6 months+ use .2% dilution (1 drop in 200 ml of carrier oil) and .5% ages 15 months+ (1 drop in 100 ml of carrier).

2%: Daily use by adults (minus daily products that were mentioned previously), occasional use in kids ages 2-6. This is still a low dilution; however, this is not recommended for anyone under the age of 2 or during pregnancy, except for sparing use in much-needed situations and with professional recommendation.

3%: Daily/occasional use by adults. I don't recommend making daily products this high of a dilution. Do not use this dilution during pregnancy, and only use with children ages 2+ and the elderly for singular uses or for serious issues. This can be used in products that might be used daily/every other day, like balms or even lotions, but not for daily care products such as deodorant or facial products that are used often during the day or on sensitive areas (like the face or underarms).

5%: Short term use by healthy adults. Not recommended for kids, the elderly, or during pregnancy. Again, this is for short term use only when addressing issues that require a higher dilution, such as pain. Do not use daily. Take breaks and discontinue use after a while. I use this dilution for things like pain balms, which I don't use daily, much like how Icy Hot is used on occasion, or pain medications are taken only occasionally. You can use this dilution daily for 1-2 weeks, and then discontinue use and take a break.

10%: This is one of the highest dilutions recommended and is strictly for singular or short-term use. Use this for extreme issues such as pulled muscles, fungal issues, etc. Do not use this dilution longer than 1 week at a time and leave breaks in between before starting this dilution again. Never use a dilution this high with children, the elderly, sick, or during pregnancy. Also avoid this dilution if breastfeeding. This is really for one time use, not for an extended period of time, and is good for pulled muscles or short-term pain/emotional relief.

Sometimes you might need higher dilutions for short term use, talk to a professional regarding using dilutions higher than 10%. They can help guide you in the best course of action and help ensure your safety.

What can you use to dilute essential oils? Things like lotions, body butters, and carrier oils (almond, grapeseed, avocado, coconut/FCO, apricot kernel, etc.) are popular choices. Carrier oils will be covered in a later chapter (Ch. 8). What you want to use is entirely up to you. For roller bottles, I recommend a liquid carrier oil, as this will yield the best results. Depending on things like individual preferences or skin type, your carrier might vary. Lotion bases and FCO (fractionated coconut oil) tend to be the most popular and inexpensive carriers.

On top of dilutions for topical use in essential oils, there are also essential oils that have a max dilution. Sometimes these max dilutions are lower than even 1% and are intended to help avoid reactions such as irritation and phototoxicity. I do not recommend ignoring these max dilutions unless instructed to do so by a professional. Even then I wouldn't recommend ignoring a topical max at all, they are in place to avoid reactions and negative effects. I have included a chart with the most popular essential oils and their topical maxes on the next page. I did not include essential oils that do not have a topical max but be sure to double-check your oil if it is not on the list. If an essential oil does not have a topical max, you still need to dilute the essential oil for topical use.

Essential oils are powerful and highly concentrated. It is worth repeating that even if you see a lot of people online telling you that, because they are natural, they're 100% safe, this is a myth. It is bad advice, and potentially dangerous. Some essential oils are more irritating, some are phototoxic (they will have a reaction in the sun), and even if some are generally non-irritating, they can still pose a threat and provoke a reaction if used undiluted. Some essential oils need to be used with special considerations as well, such as medical interactions or reasons to avoid using an oil. I will go over this more in a later chapter (Ch. 12). It is very important to know if the essential oil that you are using is one of these.

If you don't dilute an essential oil, you can become sensitized, have an allergic reaction, or just become irritated by it. One time, I used tea tree essential oil neat (undiluted) on my skin. I got a reaction and it discolored part of my skin. Diluting helps keep you safe and doesn't waste your essential oils. As essential oils are expensive, diluting can help stretch the bottle of oil and save money.

Most essential oil companies also sell high quality carrier oils but acquiring them can be as simple as going to the grocery store and picking up a bottle of olive/avocado oil. Choosing a carrier oil can also depend on what you want as far as therapeutic benefits goes. If you want your oils to be absorbed more quickly by your skin, you want to choose something like FCO (fractionated coconut oil) which is a lighter oil and more readily absorbed. You also might want something a little heavier or more moisturizing, in which case opting for something heavier might be the way to go. We will discuss the most popular carrier oils and their benefits in a later chapter (Ch. 8).

Diluting might seem intimidating, but once you get the basics it's actually really easy. Most people only use 1 or 2 different carrier oils, or lotion bases, and they are happy with what they have. Some charts might also seem confusing because they use "half" drops of essential oil. This is because drops are not the most accurate way to measure, they are just the easiest. I tend to just go down in drops if a recipe calls for half drops. So, if a dilution called for 4.5 drops, I would do 4 drops. This makes things easier, since we can't exactly measure a half drop! It also ensures that I am not going over the dilution rate stated. Better to use a little less than too much in my opinion.

ESSENTIAL OIL
TOPICAL MAXES

- *Basil linalool (Ocimum basilicum): 3.3%
- *Bergatmot (Citrus bergamia): .4%
- *Cassia (Cinnamomum cassia, Cinamomum aromatium): .05%
- *Cinnamon Bark (Cinnamomum verum, Cinnamomum zeylanicm): .01%
- *Cinamon Leaf (Cinnamomum verum, Cinnamomum zeylanicum): .06%
- *Grapefruit (Citrus paradisi): 4%

- *Jasmine (Jasminum grandiflorum, Jasminum offficinale): .7%
- *Spanish Lavender (Lavandula stoechas): 8%
- *Spike Lavender (Lavandula latifolia, Lavandula spica): 19%
- *Lemon (Citrus limon): 2%
- *Lemongrass (Cymbopogon flexuosus): .7%
- *Lime (Citrus x aurantifolia): 2%

- *Citronella (Cymbopogon winterianus, Cymbopogon nardus): 18.2%
- *Clove (Eugenia caryophyllata, Syzygium aromaticum, Eugenia aromatium): .5%
- *Eucalyptus (Globulus, Radiata): 20%
- *Geranium (Pelarganium graveolens, Pelaganium x asperum): 17.5%
- *Melissa (Melissa officinalis): .9%

- *Oregano (Origanum vulgare): 1.1%
- *Peppermint (Mentha piperita): 5.4%
- *Rosemary t Camphor (Rosmarinus offiicinalis): 16.5%
- *East indian Sandalwood (Santum album): 2%
- *Spearmint (Mentha spicata): 1.7%
- *Tea Tree (Melaleuca alternifolia): 15%
- Vetiver (Vetiveria zizanoides): 15%
- Ylang ylang (Canaga odorata): .7%

CHAPTER 7: INGESTION AND REACTIONS

This will probably be one of the shortest chapters, because I am not trained in ingestion and therefore cannot guide you through it. I also do not want to ever give this kind of guidance in a book where my words could be taken out of context or misconstrued. While in theory I know how to do this safely, I cannot (and will not) give that advice. Instead, I want to talk about why we don't casually ingest essential oils or use them as a supplement. I know that many people recommend doing so, even some aromatherapists, but ingestion is something I believe needs to be done under the supervision of a professional. It has its time and place, but the majority of people who ingest essential oils today do so in very unsafe ways.

First, essential oils are not a dietary supplement; they hold no nutritional value and are not usually beneficial to take daily. They aren't going to perk up or boost your immune system. While some essential oils contain antibacterial properties, this does not mean they are meant to be taken as a daily supplement. Their antibacterial properties are more for germ killing/fighting rather than boosting the immune system. Boosting your immune system is also a myth - that's called an autoimmune disease. But there are ways to support your immune system. So, while the use of essential oils can help in that sense, by fighting off or killing germs, they might not be benefiting you if you ingest them daily. It is best to work with a trained professional to see if ingestion would be beneficial for you and find a regimen that can be followed safely.

Secondly, since they are so highly concentrated, ingesting essential oils—especially daily—can lead to some adverse effects such as allergic reactions, sensitivities, and even in some cases organ failure. On top of that, the way that most people take essential oils does not include first properly diluting them to ensure they don't irritate any of the digestive tract on their way down. Essential oils do not mix with water, so adding essential oils to water and/or taking them directly in your mouth can cause terrible reactions and be harmful. The mouth is delicate, and subject to irritation and burns from essential oils.

Some companies will say that you can ingest their essential oils because they are so "pure", but this is not the case. The reason that you shouldn't ingest essential oils isn't because some aren't as pure, but rather because the chemical makeup of the essential oil is so concentrated. Essential oils are the essence of the plant, ten times over, and because they are so highly concentrated, they are more prone to cause irritations and reactions. Think of it this way - if you were to drink a root beer, would you want the actual drink, or just the concentrate? The base of the drink is mostly water, and the flavoring and actual soda part is about 1-2 tbsp in total. Would you enjoy 2 tbsp of root beer concentrate? Is that what you are looking for in a root beer? I have tried root beer concentrate. It's gross. Essential oils are kind of the same, except they can't be diluted in water. They are the concentrate of the plant. For example, 1 drop of peppermint essential oil is enough for around 20 cups of tea! That's a lot.

Save ingestion for when it is really needed (it's usually not) and only do so with professional help. While there is a time and place for ingestion, casual ingestion on a daily basis is certainly not it. Many companies lie about appropriate uses of their oils so that they can sell more. Don't fall for deceptive marketing tactics.

It's also important to note that ingesting essential oils by mouth might not be as beneficial as people think. They must go through your digestive tract before they can be processed by the liver. This is hard on the liver, even if you ingest in a way that is fully diluting the essential oil, and this can also process a lot less of the essential oil and give you fewer benefits.

Your stomach acid will also break down essential oils significantly, making them a little less effective when ingested. It might not be the best idea to take essential oils orally if you are expecting that method to be more powerful or helpful.

WHAT TO DO IN CASE OF REACTIONS:

Adverse reactions can and do occur with essential oils. These can include, just like with anything else, allergic reactions. This could just be a regular allergic reaction or a result of improperly using essential oils. Most of the time, reactions are the result of improper use or overuse. Either way, it is important to know how to handle a reaction.

Discontinue the use of essential oils once a reaction starts. Reactions could be a headache, rash etc. Basically, anything that happens that is abnormal to you and occurs sometime after using essential oils qualifies as a reaction. If you have a rash from topical use, gently wash the area with mild soap and warm water. You can gently rub off any remaining oil with a carrier oil as well. Rashes are NOT your body detoxing. This is a myth. If you get a rash, stop using essential oils immediately.

It is important to patch test essential oils to find out if you are allergic to them or not, especially new oils and especially if you already have allergies. Do this by mixing a 1% (.2% under 2 years of age) dilution of the oil in a carrier and applying it to the inside of your elbow. Allow to rest for 20 minutes, or up to 24/48 hours (you can cover with a bandage to keep the area protected) and see if you have any kind of reaction. If there is a reaction, do not use the essential oil in question and wash the area. If there is no reaction, you can continue to use the oil. Most people can use most essential oils, when properly diluted, and be fine. Just like with anything else, reactions can happen at other times as well.

A lot of reactions occur with excessive use, overuse, not diluting essential oils, using too much, and ingesting them excessively. Following safety guidelines will give you the best experience with essential oils. Even if you do not have a reaction to essential oils at first, using them in unsafe manners (such as not diluting or ingesting improperly) can cause sensitization that will lead to one, or lifelong allergies. It is much better to be safe. You can also have reactions in response to diffusing, although this is less common, and the same rules apply. Stop using them immediately. Make sure not to overuse a diffuser or put too many drops in.

CHAPTER 8: CARRIER OILS AND EMULSIFIERS

You may have heard the term "carrier oil" and wondered what it means. We have discussed them in a previous chapter briefly, and so maybe you already know what carrier oils are but are unsure which one is best. You always hear recommendations, but sometimes what someone else likes might not be what works for you. It also depends on what you want to use essential oils for. For example, if you want to make something for your hair, a lighter carrier oil might be preferable. But let's say you have dry skin or eczema, in which case certain carrier oils might be more beneficial. Then it gets a little more complicated if you are looking to use specific essential oils for skin care, because then you will want to pick a carrier oil that works with your skin type.

There are often recommendations to only use FCO (fractionated coconut oil) or a mix of oils that a preferred company sells. But hold up! Beyond the recommendation of "this is cheap" and "my company sells this", how can you be sure you are picking the best carrier oil for topical use? Which one is best for your skin type? What benefits do certain carriers have? Which ones is best to use? There isn't an easy answer to these questions, but we can look at each carrier oil profile and see which one you would prefer to use personally. I have put together this chapter on carrier oils and some of their best features to help. I have also listed places you can buy these carrier oils to make things easier. While I will remain brandless on essential oil preferences, I can definitely make suggestions for carrier oils.

CARRIER OILS

ALMOND OIL:
- Thicker, allows for slower absorption
- Calming, may enhance effects of some essential oils
- Soothing to inflamed skin/skin peeling from burns
- Relieves itching
- Helpful for dry skin
- Shelf life: 12 months
- Where to buy?

Plant Therapy
Simply Earth

APRICOT KERNEL OIL:
- Thinner, faster absorption
- Nourishing to the skin
- Relieves itchy skin
- Ideal for lotions
- Good for dry skin

- Shelf life: 6-12 months
- Where to buy?

Plant Therapy

ARGAN OIL:
- Vitamin E levels are high
- Has anti-aging properties
- Good in hair care, helpful to dry/frizzy hair
- Great choice for skin care, with rejuvenating and regenerating properties
- Popular oil in commercial hair care
- Shelf life: 24 months (about 2 years)
- Where to buy?

Plant Therapy

AVOCADO OIL:
- Useful for inflamed skin
- May help prevent premature aging
- Highly moisturizing
- Refrigeration can change the consistency of this oil
- Popular oil due to its fatty content, nice choice for lotions and body butters
- Shelf life: 12 months
- Where to buy?

Plant Therapy
Simply Earth

COCONUT OIL/FCO:
- Makes a great massage oil
- Nourishing to hair/scalp; ideal for hair masks
- Often used in suppositories because of its ability to become solid and remelt
- Helps soaps lather
- Antibacterial properties make it a favorite choice for oil pulling and oral health
- Absorbs a little more readily than other oils
- Shelf life of coconut oil: about 2-4 years, FCO can last indefinitely
- Where to buy?

Plant Therapy (FCO)
Simply Earth (Coconut)
Simply Earth (FCO)

GRAPESEED OIL:
- Versatile oil, used for most skin types
- Ideal for the skin, soothing and regenerative
- Hypoallergenic, making it an ideal choice even for sensitive people
- Less greasy than other oils
- Absorbs the fastest
- Shelf life: 3-6 months, up to 9 months in the fridge
- Where to buy?

Plant Therapy

JOJOBA:
- This is technically a wax
- Anti-inflammatory
- Ideal choice for dry skin conditions
- Composition of the oil is similar to the skin's natural oil (sebum)
- Despite being thicker, this oil isn't very greasy
- Shelf life: indefinitely
- Where to buy?

Plant Therapy
Simply Earth

MEADOWFOAM OIL:
- Stable shelf life
- Can penetrate skin easier than other oils
- May delay aging and wrinkles
- Holds up better under heat, ideal for DIYs
- Ideal and versatile as an ingredient for things like lotions, body butters, etc.
- Shelf life: Indefinite
- Where to buy?

Plant Therapy
Simply Earth

OLIVE OIL:
- Anti-inflammatory and soothing to the skin (may aggravate dandruff)
- May work as pain relief, ideal for blending with pain relieving essential oils
- Anti-aging properties
- Good for treating bruising
- Shelf life: 12-18 months
- Where to buy?

Aromatics international

ROSEHIP OIL:
- Excellent skin oil and very popular for topical use
- Ideal for addressing scarring due to regenerative properties
- Useful for healing wounds and burns
- Can help improve eczema and acne
- Beneficial to aging skin
- Very low shelf life, this oil is subject to spoilage
- Shelf life: 6 months
- Where to buy?

Plant Therapy

SESAME OIL:
- Antioxidant
- Helpful in repairing eczema and psoriasis
- Useful in treating lice
- Soothing to the digestive tract when used internally

- Shelf life: 6-9 months, up to a year in the fridge
- Where to buy?

Mountain Rose Herbs

TAMANU OIL:
- Antibacterial; often used for acne, blemishes, and fungal infections
- Soothing anti-inflammatory properties
- Good choice for healing appearance of scars
- Useful oil for treating pain
- Shelf life: 12-24 months (about 2 years)
- Where to buy:

Aromatics International

TRAUMA OIL:
- This is an herbal blend oil (in olive oil) that you can make or buy
- Great for all kinds of topical skin issues
- Good to use for bumps, bruising, cuts, scrapes etc. (please note trauma oil contains arnica which should not be applied to open wounds as arnica is poison to the blood; apply around a cut or scrape to promote healing and reduce inflammation but do not apply directly to the open wound)
- Can help with swelling and inflammation
- Shelf life: Will last as long as the carrier used, commonly olive oil is used
- Where to buy:

Make your own (Ch. 13) or purchase a premade blend, many herbal and aromatherapy companies sell their own.

There are several other carriers that can be used to make products containing essential oils such as beeswax, shea butter, mango butter, cocoa butter, or even a store-bought unscented lotion base. Many butters are ideal for dry skin. These all count as carriers; while not strictly defined as "oil" themselves, they will do the job of diluting essential oils for topical use. This also means making an array of naturally scented products with essential oils is much easier than it seems.

WHAT DOESN'T COUNT AS A CARRIER OIL?

It is commonly recommended to use something that isn't actually considered a carrier oil and therefore won't properly mix with the essential oils. It's important to know which oils are appropriate for diluting and which ones are not so great.

ALOE VERA:

This is often used as a carrier for things like burns/sunburn, but since aloe is water based it makes for a less-than-ideal carrier. There needs to be a thickener in the aloe to make this an appropriate carrier, and most aloe on the market is not commercially thickened. This isn't an inherently bad thing, because it has many uses beyond aromatherapy and doesn't need to be thickened, but it is not so good when someone shares their DIY sunburn relief, and they use a watery aloe vera gel. Don't be fooled by the word "gel", this substance is anything but thick when it comes to using it as a carrier for essential oils. Plant Therapy does offer a thickened aloe jelly that is perfect for your aromatherapy DIYs, and this would be fine to use. Unless it specifies that the aloe vera is thickened, it is not appropriate to use as a base for essential oils and it does not work to combine the oils properly.

VITAMIN E:

While technically dubbed an oil, this is a vitamin and doesn't properly mix with essential oils. You can use this in recipes with another carrier oil, but by itself it does not make a good carrier.

WITCH HAZEL:

Despite being widely regarded as an emulsifier for liquid-based products, this is not the case. Witch hazel should not be used as the base for applying essential oils topically. Either use an emulsifier (something that helps essential oils bind to a liquid) or just a carrier oil. You can find a natural emulsifier/solubilizer online for your water-based DIYs.

EMULSIFIERS

You've probably heard this word and then either wondered what it means, or you know what it means but aren't sure what constitutes an emulsifier or why someone would even need one. So, what are emulsifiers, how do they pertain to essential oils/aromatherapy, and why do you need them?

"Emulsifier: Emulsifiers, in foods and beauty products, are any number of chemical additives that encourage the suspension of one liquid in another. Emulsifiers are closely related to stabilizers, which are substances that maintain the emulsified state. Emulsifiers, stabilizers, and related compounds are also used in the preparation of cosmetics, lotions, and certain pharmaceuticals, where they serve much the same purpose as in foods- i.e., they prevent separation of ingredients and extend storage life." (Britannica, The Editors of Encyclopaedia. "emulsifier". Encyclopedia Britannica, 9 Apr. 2021, https://www.britannica.com/science/emulsifier. Accessed 4 July 2024.)

Emulsification is essentially a fancy way of saying we are blending an oil into another liquid well enough that the two substances do not separate. But why is this important? Essential oils do not mix with water, at least not well. Most essential oils will float on the surface of water, and while others might mix for a time or sink to the bottom (depending on the density of the oil) they will never truly mix into water or most other liquids. So, if you are wanting to use an essential oil topically in any kind of water-based product (like a perfume or room spray), you will want (and need) an emulsifier/binder/stabilizer to make that happen. The reason you want to mix your essential oils in a water-based product with an emulsifier is because otherwise when you use the product essential oils will separate and then can cause reactions or be unsafe when, eventually, neat and undiluted essential oil hits your skin. Using an emulsifier ensures that the essential oil is totally mixed into the product and won't be leaving any undiluted essential oils in the product.

It is important to note that while I use the words "emulsifier" and "emulsion", this is not always what happens when mixing essential oils with a water base; most often the essential oils are broken down or bound with another chemical/product that will then mix into water. I know that emulsifier is not technically the correct term to use here, but it is the best one to explain what is going on, because we are indeed working to mix essential oils with water-based items. Solubilizer or solubilizing is another word that can describe what happens when we bind essential oils (or dissolve/mix them) into a liquid base.

So then, what makes an emulsifier? What are some products that will bind or dissolve essential oils into a water-based solution and make them safe to use? When do you need to be using an emulsifier?

MAKING THE EMULSION

An emulsifier is basically any product that suspends one liquid (or substance) in another. Eggs are emulsifiers when you are making mayonnaise. You wouldn't use an egg for essential oils, of course-I hope! And it's slightly different when working with essential oils because they aren't the exact same as water, but they aren't really an oil either despite being called one. In the aromatherapy world, we have a few things that would work as an emulsifier, and many more that are commonly thought to be one but really aren't.

EMULSIFIERS TO USE

- **BEESWAX/CANDELILLA:** Waxes acts as an emulsifier in lotions. Beeswax is the most common but candelilla is the vegan option. While you can use essential oils in an unscented lotion base that has already been made, you need something in the lotion if you are making it. As lotion consists mostly of water, the wax acts as the emulsifier when combining water with the oils. You can add essential oils to the oil portion and then make your lotion, or simply make the lotion and then add oils. I personally prefer to make my lotion first and then add oils. Using wax can be a little tricky though, as you must melt it down with any other oil you are using before adding it (once cooled slightly) to the water in a blender (a little at a time) and then blend like crazy! Most people end up buying a lotion base. It is much easier to get a good base and add the essential oils to that. Some people also say that beeswax or candelilla wax are not emulsifiers, which is false. I don't know where this myth stemmed from, but most waxes are recognized as emulsifiers or are acknowledged as being able to create an emulsion when combined with other ingredients. If you are making a lotion base, follow the recipe correctly (also have a good recipe) so that nothing goes wrong. It is easy to tell if a lotion is off, so you will know if it's not mixed correctly.
- **ALCOHOL:** This one is a little trickier. Through trial and error, I found that you need a incredibly high proof of alcohol for this to work. Even then, it's not that great. I use Everclear, which is about 190 proof. I use this for things like sprays, where the base is entirely water. It's not my favorite method, and again it's not perfect. I have found that using anything with a lower proof is not going to

result in a proper mix. The recommended minimum for using alcohol is 150 proof. The reason that alcohol works is that it will break down and disperse the essential oils. So, while this isn't classified as a true emulsion process, for the purpose of this book it's the word I will use because it most closely represents what is happening since the alcohol works to mix the essential oils in a water base.

- **POLYSORBATE 20:** Polysorbate 20 is a synthetic emulsifier, derived from polyethoxylated sorbitan and oleic acid. This one is controversial because it is synthetic, designed to emulate the fatty acids from animals and vegetables. While initially derived from natural sources, it is changed so thoroughly that it qualifies as a synthetic product. I used to use this before realizing it was synthetic and have now found other sources I prefer to use. But if you don't mind synthetic, this is a great option. Polysorbate 20 works by breaking down the oils (much like alcohol, but more efficiently) and thus making them able to be mixed into liquids. It is the most popular emulsifier on the market, appearing in a wide variety of products from skincare to food items. You may see polysorbate on packaging as polysorbate 80 or polysorbate 20. For the purpose of mixing with essential oils, stick with polysorbate 20.
- **CASTILE LIQUID SOAP/BUBBLE BATH/LIQUID SOAP BASE:** This can work as an "emulsifier" of sorts (although what is actually happening is better defined as solubilization more than anything) IF you mix oils into the soap base before mixing this with the liquid. You will often see someone mix the entire DIY mixture into water and then add oils after the fact. This will not properly mix the essential oil into the liquids. When you hear that castile soap can work as an emulsifier of sorts, you might not think the order matters when mixing the ingredients. But it really does matter. It will make for a much cleaner DIY when mixed properly. I have never had any separation issues when mixing essential oils into castile soap first.
- **NATURAL SOLUBILIZER:** This is my favorite for emulsification, as it is an all-natural emulsifier that helps to bind essential oils to water. This product is the natural version of polysorbate. It consists of caprylyl capryl glucoside, and not that I generally place much weight on this, but caprylyl capryl glucoside scored a 2 on the EWG website. As far as options go, this is one of the best ones from an all-natural standpoint. You can find caprylyl capryl glucoside in many places, simply search for it and options to purchase pop up, ranging from small bottles to bulk buying options. I know some people would still find issues with this product, and that is fine. We need to think of the importance of safety in this instance though, and the benefits of this product far outweigh any negatives there might be for the sake of safely emulsifying essential oils.

WHEN TO USE EMULSIFIERS

Anytime essential oils don't mix and incorporate into a product on their own, you need to use an emulsifier. This is generally with water-based products but, like I mentioned before, if the product is already made and has an emulsifier present (like lotion) then you can safely add essential oils. Things like room sprays would need an emulsifier. Bath salts/bath bombs would also need an emulsifier or a carrier oil, as you will be using the product in the bath and essential oils don't mix with bath water. Using a carrier oil in the bath will make the tub slippery though so be aware of that. Also, if you want to use essential oils topically with a water-based product (such as a perfume), they need to be diluted with a carrier oil or properly emulsified product. You do not need one if the "liquid" in question is an oil (however vitamin E oil doesn't count as a carrier oil, as previously discussed), if the product is already emulsified (like a lotion base), or if the product doesn't contain water/water-based liquids. Essential oils mix with carrier oils and butters (shea, cocoa, or mango) so you don't need anything extra to mix the product.

COMMON ITEMS THOUGHT TO BE EMULSIFIERS

Misinformation when it comes to what people think are emulsifiers is often shared online, however unless it completely mixes the oils it's not a true emulsifier and is still leaving undiluted essential oil throughout a product.

- **WITCH HAZEL:** Many people claim that this works in room sprays and hair sprays to emulsify essential oils, but it actually doesn't. The oils float on the top of the witch hazel and put you at risk for coming into contact with undiluted essential oils when you use the product. As discussed earlier, witch hazel alone isn't enough to dilute or emulsify essential oils.
- **SALT:** While salt is technically an emulsifier, at least according to Google, it doesn't really work (at least it never has for me), especially in larger dilutions with essential oils. You might have seen people add essential oils to bath salts, or use salt in a room spray, and this can (technically) work, but for the sake of safety I am adding this to the no list because I have also seen this go wrong. It can be pretty finicky. Having undiluted essential oils floating around your bath is not ideal, nor is having a room spray that doesn't properly mix with its water base. I believe that you need a certain type of salt for this to work. Quite honestly, I tried this myself and was less than pleased with the result and so didn't pursue it any further. It is also going out of "style" so to say that you can use salts as a carrier, I know this used to pretty popular, but the latest research is showing that this isn't safe to do as salt is water soluble.
- **MILK:** Milk was thought to work as an emulsifier or carrier of sorts for essential oils, but this is no longer accepted in the aromatherapy world. As research progresses, so does knowledge. Milk used to be much fattier, but modern pasteurizing methods have removed most of the fat. The idea was that milk was fatty, like an oil, that you could use it. This is no longer the case with modern milk production and milk is unsafe to use in this manner.
- **VINEGAR:** Vinegar is yet another that is assumed to disperse essential oils. Vinegar needs to be more powerful, though. I have also tried this one, and I let the essential oils sit for a month. They remained floating on top of the vinegar after a whole month. I know many people love to make homemade cleaners and add essential oils; I don't necessarily hate this, especially if you use a rag and gloves to clean. But you can also just steep some herbs or orange peels in the vinegar for a month and get the same effect.

- **ALCOHOLS:** Like I mentioned before, unless you have a high enough proof of alcohol, it's just not going to work. You really must have the highest proof of alcohol (190 proof or 95% alcohol) and you can't use rubbing alcohol, because it generally does not reach a high enough proof. A lot of DIY recipes call for vodka or rubbing alcohol, and this is simply misleading advice because it is not strong enough to be able to work as some people claim. Alcohol is also a popular choice of preservative, but again you need a high enough proof for that (120 proof for use as a preservative) so it's really important to make sure you have the right kind of alcohol, or it won't work. Ethanol, Everclear, and perfumer's alcohol are popular choices with a high enough proof. I personally no longer use alcohol because you need such a high proof, and it can be fairly unreliable.
- **ALOE VERA:** While a popular choice for DIYs and emulsification, aloe vera gel is a water-based substance and does not actually mix with the essential oils. It gives the impression that it does, seeming to mix a lot better than water or witch hazel, but it does not. Plant Therapy has an aloe vera jelly that comes thickened, which is better suited for our purposes and comes ready to add essential oils to. This is the only exception that I know of, and you will otherwise need something else to mix in with aloe to be able to make it work. As previously discussed, this just doesn't work with essential oils.

USING EMULSIFIERS

So, we know what emulsifiers are, but how do we use them? For things like beeswax/candelilla, it's best to follow a good lotion recipe and then add the essential oils to the finished product. I have found this works best and is relatively easy to do once you get the hang of making a lotion, or if you buy a lotion base it becomes even easier. How do things like alcohol, natural solubilizers, and polysorbates work? With alcohol, you will determine the allotted amount for your recipe, measure it out, and then add the amount of essential oil that you want. You need to let this sit, so it is best to do this in a separate container. This could take some time. It often requires 15-20 minutes, maybe even longer if the density of the oil is heavier. Once the oils have degraded down and you can mix them into the alcohol and they don't settle back at the top, you are good to go. Continue with the recipe as stated. With a solubilizer or polysorbate, you will add them in addition to the recipe. Polysorbate is a 2:1 ratio, and solubilizer a 3:1 ratio. For polysorbate, you will do 2 parts of the polysorbate and 1-part essential oil. With the solubilizer, it's 3 parts solubilizer and 1-part essential oil. You will then let them sit for around 15-20 minutes, although this time can vary depending on the density of the essential oils being used. Once it has settled, gently swirl or stir and then add to your DIY as you add the essential oils and mix gently. Your product is now properly combined and will last longer without separation.

When mixing essential oils with castile soap, all that you need to do is thoroughly mix the oils and soap base together. Once you have done this, you can continue with the DIY project as you normally would, adding the allotted amount of water, oils, glycerin etc.

Hopefully this provided some insight on emulsifiers and what to look for to ensure your products are properly formulated. This can also be helpful when checking a product you are considering buying. If you see it is water-based and you don't see an emulsifier, I recommend taking caution with that product.

Now this is certainly not an extensive list. I left out some of the more unknown or uncommon ones, but it will give you a general idea of carrier oils and emulsifiers and which ones would be best for you based on their benefits, properties, and shelf lives. Hopefully this helps and can shed some light on all the different carrier oils and emulsifiers out there.

When storing; always make sure to store essential oils, carrier oils, and emulsifiers in a cool, dry, and dark location. Avoid UV rays and heat as these things can degrade or break down the product faster. The same goes for storing products made with essential oils. Some things last longer in the fridge, however some shouldn't be put in the fridge. Always make sure to check your products for spoilage; any cloudiness/discoloration or change in scent/taste (if you can taste the item) means the product has gone bad and should be tossed out. Hopefully this chapter is helpful when it comes to making essential oil products or formulating your DIY projects.

CHAPTER 9: USING ESSENTIAL OILS WHILE PREGNANT OR BREASTFEEDING

This chapter will be quite lengthy and broken into different sections (clinical and non-clinical). There's a lot to cover with pregnancy and breastfeeding, as well as some other things to consider when essential oils are used by this population. There are a few questions to ask when thinking about using essential oils in pregnancy. Do you want to adhere to the strict clinical studies and rules regarding pregnancy? Do you care if an essential oil is considered safe but hasn't been studied in a clinical setting? Do you feel comfortable using essential oils at all? These are some of the questions to ask yourself before using essential oils while pregnant or breastfeeding. I will be talking about general use of aromatherapy in pregnancy, as well as clinical aromatherapy in pregnancy. To be clear, clinical aromatherapy is something I am not certified in yet although I have extensively studied it. I have learned through my courses and first-hand knowledge what is considered clinically safe in pregnancy, and I can share the information regarding clinically studied essential oils that already exists. I am currently working towards my clinical certification but am not certified yet so please exercise your own due diligence and know what is regarded as safe with the current research available. This chapter will also be a little repetitive as I have designed it to be skimmed over and be jumped around in for reference use, I know that some people will want to reference clinical vs non-clinical or that they won't read this chapter in its entirety. For the sake of safety, this chapter is specifically designed to look (and repeat) a certain way for referencing.

A crucial thing to remember with pregnancy is that the main concern lies in the potential for essential oils to cross the placenta to the baby. It is believed that this does happen, and therefore there are certain guidelines to adhere to. The same thing goes for breastfeeding - it is believed that some can make their way into the milk, and therefore into the baby. Caution and safety is always advised here.

ARE ESSENTIAL OILS SAFE TO USE DURING PREGNANCY?

Oftentimes people claim that essential oils are 100% safe in pregnancy, and that there are no rules to abide by, because they are natural and that makes them categorically safe. Well, just because something is natural does not make it safe! And there are actually a lot of guidelines to using essential oils in pregnancy. Many essential oils are not safe, and the ones that are safe still come with cautions, especially regarding pregnancy. In this chapter I will detail in depth what essential oils are safe, what essential oils aren't safe (and need to be avoided), rules and guidelines for using essential oils during pregnancy, and some ways we can utilize essential oils during pregnancy/labor. First, let's go over some basics on essential oil usage during pregnancy.

The general consensus across the board is that, yes, essential oil usage is safe in pregnancy and does not pose much of a risk. I find this to be a pretty broad statement, and just because something is generally safe does not always make it safe for all individuals. Some things to consider before using essential oils during pregnancy are: What trimester of pregnancy are you in? Is your pregnancy high risk? Does your care provider know and approve of using essential oils during your pregnancy? Are the oils you are wanting to use pregnancy-safe, classified as safe to use, and without toxicity risk to you or your baby? Are you on medications that could interact with essential oils?

Generally speaking, a lot of essential oils are fine to use during pregnancy, meaning they don't pose any risks. But that is, once again, a broad statement. As helpful as it is to know which oils are widely considered to be safe, this does not dive into the complexities of using essential oils while pregnant. There actually haven't been a lot of studies on essential oil usage during pregnancy, and honestly what studies have been done involved rats or other animals and not humans. This might be enough for you, or it might not be. I find myself on the fence. Rat testing can yield similar results to what would happen in human trials, but a human trial would provide the best and most accurate information. While we can evaluate the chemical make-up of essential oils and perform animal testing, this can only tell us so much about how an essential oil would react in someone who is pregnant.

There are not a ton of studies, which also means that there aren't any reported cases of essential oils causing any issues in pregnancy, either from lack of studies or lack of evidence. However, there are definitely essential oils to avoid, due to their chemical constituents. These are generally common knowledge, although some advice from certain companies or untrained sources might say otherwise. So, here is the list of essential oils that should never be used during pregnancy, and need to be avoided at all costs topically, aromatically, and internally.

ESSENTIAL OILS TO AVOID (NEVER USE) DURING PREGNANCY:
- Anise *Pimpinella anisum*
- Anise star *Illicium verum*
- Arborvitae *Thuja plicata*
- Birch (sweet) *Betula lenta*
- Black seed *Nigella sativa*
- Buchu (diosphenol CT and pulegone CT) *Agathosma betulina, Agathosm cenulata*
- Camphor (brown) *Cinnamomum camphora*
- Carrot seed *Daucus carota*
- Cassia *Cinnamomum cassia, Cinnamomum aromaticum*
- Chaste tree *Vitex agnus castus*
- Cinnamon bark *Cinnamomum verum/Cinnamomum zeylanicum*
- Costus *Saussurea costus*
- Cypress (blue) *Callitris intratopica*
- Dill seed (Indian) *Anthem sowa*
- Fennel (bitter and sweet) *Foeniculum vulgare*
- Ho leaf (camphor CT) *Cinnamomum camphora ct camphor*

- Hyssop (pinocamphine CT) *Hssopus officinalis ct pinocamphine*
- Lavender (spanish) *Lavandula stoechas*
- Mugwort (common/camphor/thujone CT, common chrysanthenyl acetate CT and great) *Artemisia vulgaris ct camphor/thujone, Artemisia vulgaris ct chrysanthemum acetate, Artemisia arborescens*
- Myrrh *Commiphora myrrha, Commiphora molmol*
- Myrtle *Myrtus communis, Melaleuca tererifolia, Backhousia citriodora*
- Nutmeg *Myristica fragrans, Myristica officinalis, Myristica moschata, Myristica aromatica, Myristica amboinensis*
- Oregano *Origanum vulgare, Origanum onites*
- Parsley *Cymbopogon martinii, Adropogon martinii*
- Pennyroyal *Hedeoma pulegioides, Mentha pulegium, Micromeria fruticosa*
- Rue *Ruta graveolens, Ruta montana*
- Sage (dalmatian and Spanish) *Salvia officinalis, Salvia lavandulifolia, Salvia hispanorum*
- Tansy *Tanacetum vulgare, Chrysanthemum tanacetum*
- Tea tree (black) *Melaleuca bracteata*
- Wintergreen *Gaultheria procumbens, Gaultheria fragrantissima*

I did not include every single oil, because a lot of them are uncommon and not even sold. Even some on this list are little known in the aromatherapy world. However, a few of them are common and widely sold, and even recommended to pregnant women all the time, such as wintergreen, cassia, and cinnamon bark, among others. The reasoning for avoiding these oils is that they hold the most risk and can cause issues for a mother and her pregnancy, such as being:

- Neurotoxic: causes destruction of nerve tissue
- Carcinogenic: causes cancer
- Hepatotoxic: toxic to the liver
- Nephrotoxic: toxic to the kidneys
- Abortifacient: causes abortion/terminates pregnancy
- Embryotoxic: toxic to the baby growing in utero (specifically in the first 8 weeks of gestation)
- Fetotoxic: toxic to the growing baby in utero
- Teratogenic: ability to cause malformations in a growing baby

At best, nothing happens, and at worst you could lose your baby or cause some serious side effects during pregnancy. It is also important to note that utilizing essential oils and herbs to affect a pregnancy in anyway is not recommended to do. I know popular advice was floating around on herbs or essential oils that could terminate a pregnancy, but this is not something to attempt at home as it could end very badly or cause you harm-even death. Aromatherapists and herbalists caution against this and don't recommend trying to do so, or even sharing advice to try and do so.

Now let's get into how we can utilize essential oils during pregnancy, and how aromatherapy can help with a pregnancy. Some things to remember and consider when using essential oils during pregnancy are:

- Avoid essential oils as much as possible in the first trimester
- Respect topical maxes of all essential oils, and remember to never go above a .5%-1% dilution in pregnancy
- NEVER ingest essential oils during pregnancy, even if the oil is safe for pregnancy
- Use essential oils moderately and appropriately throughout the entire pregnancy

NEVER use an essential oil that is not pregnancy safe. Alternatively, a hydrosol is a great option to use, and you can always replace essential oils with them whenever possible. I will talk about hydrosols more in a later chapter (Ch. 10).

AVOID ESSENTIAL OILS AS MUCH AS POSSIBLE IN THE FIRST TRIMESTER: You should really limit your use of essential oils in the first trimester, ideally avoiding them all together. Advice may vary on this, but most professionals seem to agree on avoiding usage as much as possible. Do not use an essential oil unless you really need to. Sometimes aromatherapy can be beneficial for morning sickness, although I would try other methods before turning to essential oils. If you do decide to, then opt for aromatic use vs topical use and never ingest an essential oil while pregnant. I knew someone who claimed it was safe to ingest an essential oil blend containing cassia (one of the oils that is toxic in pregnancy) to help with morning sickness. Cassia essential oil is an embryotoxic oil, meaning it can be toxic to the baby growing in utero. Obviously, this is not something that should be done, no matter how "comfortable" you feel with it! With the limited studies we do have, this much is apparent, and studying the chemical makeups of essential oils can tell us if something is going to be an issue during pregnancy. Just because someone says it is safe and does it themselves, doesn't mean it is. Be wary of advice online given by people who fail to do their research. A lack of proper research on something, or a lack of negative side effects, does not mean that it is safe.

RESPECT THOSE TOPICAL MAXES: Do not exceed the topical max of 1% during pregnancy, for all oils. Some oils have a max dilution of less than that; do not exceed these. I would personally recommend keeping the dilution low. I used a .5% dilution during my pregnancy. We also want to limit how often we are using essential oils, which is something we should be doing anyways even if we aren't pregnant. Some advice out there has people using essential oils several times daily, or even up to 10x a day! This is certainly not something to be doing during pregnancy. Use sparingly, and only when necessary. Daily use 1-3x a day at a .5% dilution is a great goal. Use oils for relaxation, for morning sickness, and pregnancy pains. Utilize oils in labor, but don't go overboard on topical maxes or use oils every hour of every day! Remember it is important to give the body a break when it comes to using essential oils.

USE ESSENTIAL OILS APPROPRIATELY: Don't pump your lotion full of essential oils, don't diffuse essential oils 24 hours a day (half hour increments with 1-2 hour breaks is key), don't use oils topically every hour of every day, don't ignore dilutions, don't ingest essential oils, don't stick essential oils in your vagina (or rectum), and don't use essential oils that are unsafe to use during pregnancy.

ALTERNATIVELY, USE HYDROSOLS: For example, a peppermint hydrosol can be used to help curb nausea, or rose hydrosol can be used for skin conditions and skin soothing. I have included a list below of hydrosols, where to buy them, and what they could be good for in pregnancy. I am only listing ones I think would be beneficial in pregnancy though, so this certainly isn't an extensive list. As a reminder from earlier, hydrosols are leftover plant water from the distillation of essential oils and are a safe alternative to use during pregnancy, or with children and pets. They pose little risk and are much milder than essential oils. I will discuss hydrosols more in a later chapter (Ch. 10).

HYDROSOLS:

- Balsam fir: Congestion, achy joints
- Basil: Gas or digestive issues
- Calendula: Bumps/bruises, itchiness- Plant Therapy
- Cedarwood: itchiness
- Roman chamomile: digestive issues, itchiness, headaches, PMS- Plant Therapy
- Cinnamon bark: Gas, stimulating (coffee replacement)- Aromatics International
- Clary sage: Emotional health- Mountain Rose Herbs
- Cypress: Hemorrhoids, scars
- Eucalyptus: Congestion- Mountain Rose Herbs
- Frankincense: Skin care- Mountain Rose Herbs
- Geranium: Emotional health- Aromatics International
- Helichrysum: Scars, bumps/bruises- Mountain Rose Herbs
- Lavender: Skin care, calming, itchiness, emotional health- Simply Earth
- Neroli: Menstrual cramps (would most likely work on Braxton hicks as well)
- Peppermint: congestion, digestive issues, headaches, itchiness, nausea, stimulating- Plant Therapy
- Rose: Skin care- Simply Earth
- Rosemary: digestive issues, stimulating, thinning hair- Aromatics International
- Tea tree: Fungal issues (yeast infections, UTIs etc.)- Plant Therapy

When in doubt, use a hydrosol instead. Since hydrosols are so much milder than essential oils, they are safer to use in pregnancy. They can be ingested and used internally, so some peppermint hydrosol in your water is a better option for nausea than ingesting peppermint oil (and a peppermint tea is a much better option than ingesting the essential oil). You can safely use a hydrosol aromatically, topically, or internally during pregnancy to help with various issues. Some contraindications might still apply with specific herbs, and they do contain a small amount of the essential oil as well. While there are even less studies that I have found on hydrosols than oils during pregnancy, they are generally considered a much gentler option, especially for babies. A hydrosol can replace a lot of essential oil usage as well, making sure the amount of potential crossover of the placenta is limited. Also, please educate yourself on hydrosols a little more before ingesting or using them internally. Diluting them in water for ingestion is key in most cases, and there are important steps to take with other methods as well. I am still learning about hydrosols, so I can't speak too much on them. I highly recommend looking up trusted sources and researching this on your own. A great option is to pick up the book Hydrosols: The Next Aromatherapy by Suzanne Catty. She talks about hydrosols in much greater depth than I can, but I have included more information on hydrosols in a later chapter (Ch. 10).

A lot of the guidelines pertaining to use during pregnancy are guidelines we should all be following anyway! No one should ever go above max dilutions, ingestion is never necessary in pregnancy, and we shouldn't be using toxic essential oils. We also shouldn't be diffusing massive amounts, and we shouldn't be using essential oils more than necessary. As long your usage of essential oils is limited to an appropriate amount, you should be fine.

There is still the question of the lack of research on the safety using essential oils in pregnancy, and if essential oils cross to the placenta. Is there enough research to call this safe? Honestly, I'm not sure. People are often willing to accept essential oils because they're safer than "traditional" medicines used in pregnancy, but in actuality there are limited studies on their effects when it comes to pregnancy. Then again, there are limited studies on traditional medicines used in pregnancy as well. We are in an area that is going to be hard to judge this based off of the studies available because, in all honesty, no pregnant woman is willing to be the subject of a study that is rigorous enough to determine if there is a risk! It really just boils down to following the guidelines that we do have with essential oils, avoiding the toxic oils, and taking care during pregnancy. But look, if you are more comfortable diffusing an essential oil for morning sickness than taking a prescribed medicine, the possibility of harm from that is incredibly slim so long as you are following the guidelines that exist. Many aromatherapy books touch on the fact that proper and limited use of essential oils during pregnancy poses little risk anyway.

It's also important to note that while peppermint is considered safe during pregnancy, it isn't recommended while breastfeeding because of the potential to drop milk supply. Also, rosemary is an oil up for debate in the community, with leading aromatherapists considering it safe and other sources saying to avoid it. Generally, it is considered safe with the cineole and camphor CT, however caution should still be used with this oil. If you don't need it, don't use it. When in doubt, don't use oil.

CLINICAL AROMATHERAPY FOR PREGNANCY

In this section, I will cover the basics of clinical aromatherapy for pregnancy and go into more detail on how to utilize essential oils during pregnancy in a safe and effective way that aligns with clinical aromatherapy.

SO, WHAT IS CLINICAL AROMATHERAPY?

Clinical aromatherapy is simply aromatherapy in a hospital or clinical setting, practiced by nurses or medical professionals. This differs from other aromatherapy certifications because of the education and background involved. Nurses (and midwives) will learn about certain oils in a clinical setting as well as their therapeutic properties and methods that have been proven to be safe and effective. Clinical aromatherapists possess the understanding and medical background to apply essential oils safely to their patients. Clinical aromatherapy is also heavily backed by clinical studies and tends to be the safest (and most cautious) route. This might be the ideal choice during pregnancy, especially if you are concerned about the lack of studies regarding essential oils and pregnancy. Generally, you would seek professional help and care for clinical aromatherapy. A midwife simply selling essential oils is not a trained clinical aromatherapist, so beware of this. I know many midwives end up joining a company to sell oils and implement them into their practice. This can be unsafe as the advice from some companies isn't studied or recommended for pregnancy.

WHAT ARE SOME ESSENTIAL OILS THAT ARE CLINICALLY SAFE DURING PREGNANCY?

- First trimester: Lemon Citrus limonum
- Second Trimester: Lavender Lavandula angustifolia, lemon Citrus limonum
- Third Trimester: Bergamot Citrus bergamia, lavender Lavandula angustifolia, lemon Citrus limonum, neroli Citrus aurantium, petitgrain Citrus aurantium

These five are the only oils that have been clinically studied with those who are pregnant. I have not mentioned breastfeeding here, as I will have an entire section dedicated to it. A lot of the information for pregnancy crosses over because the main concern of essential oils crossing over to the baby is still present.

WHAT ARE THE USES OF THESE OILS DURING PREGNANCY?

- Lemon: Depression, hyperemesis, morning sickness, stress
- Lavender: Anxiety, depression, fear, pain, sleep, stress
- Bergamot: Anxiety, depression, pain, stress
- Neroli: Anxiety, depression, fear, sleep
- Petitgrain: Anxiety, depression, stress

WHAT ARE SOME WAYS TO USE ESSENTIAL OILS DURING PREGNANCY?

Since lemon is the only essential oil that has been clinically studied during the first trimester, I recommend not using essential oils at that time or only using lemon essential oil aromatically. This is my personal recommendation, though I do believe there are some cases where topical use would be beneficial. Clinically, it is recommended to avoid all essential oils until your 10th week.

INHALATION: You can diffuse, but during pregnancy our sense of smell is heightened and so it is recommended to use a personal inhaler or a cotton pad. This makes it so that if you are irritated by the scent, it won't linger, and you can quickly move it away from you. Apply a few drops (1-5 in a personal inhaler) and place just below the nose, inhaling deeply for a few seconds. Discontinue use if you have any adverse reactions such as nausea or headaches.

Alongside inhalation, making a spray is a really great way to utilize essential oils aromatically. Be aware that this method will mean that the smell lingers a little longer, like when using a diffuser. You can make a spray in a variety of ways, the simplest being with 5 ml of carrier oil in a 1oz spray bottle filled with distilled water. Add up to 12 drops of essential oil to the carrier oil and mix with water in the spray bottle. You can use aloe vera gel instead of a carrier oil, but as we have covered this doesn't fully mix/emulsify the oils and you need to make sure you have a jelly, not just aloe vera. Plant Therapy makes an aloe vera jelly that would be good for this. Alternatively, you can use an emulsifier like the one from Simply Earth (soluble) or polysorbate 20, and to make the product last longer you can use a preservative. There is a good natural preservative option available from Simply Earth as well.

TOPICALLY: You can use topically with a carrier oil or lotion base. You want to maintain a .5-1% dilution for pregnancy, and never exceed 2% (honestly, I wouldn't go above 1% unless it was seriously needed and/or later in the pregnancy). Topical use is a great option for anything past the second trimester.

Another way to use essential oils topically is in the bath. Never use essential oils neat in the bath. Always dilute them in a carrier oil before adding them to the bath. Do NOT add oils to the bath you will use during labor. Use 1-8 drops (diluted) for a bath or foot soak.

WHAT ARE SOME THINGS TO AVOID WHEN USING ESSENTIAL OILS DURING PREGNANCY?

Avoid taking advice from just anyone - ask if they are certified, and for their sources. Anyone who is a certified aromatherapist and knows their stuff will not mind sharing their sources and education. They do not have to be a clinical aromatherapist, but if you want clinical aromatherapy, I recommend seeking out someone who is clinically trained. Most people who are selling essential oils do not know what they are talking about when it comes to essential oil use during pregnancy. I certainly wouldn't take advice from anyone who recommends essential oil use in the first trimester, who recommends ingestion during pregnancy, who recommends using extremely high dilutions during pregnancy, or who says, "because it's natural it's safe."

Do not ingest essential oils during pregnancy. Absolutely no internal use of essential oils while pregnant is recommended, as it is believed that essential oils do cross over into the placenta. Using essential oils internally in any form poses a much larger risk of overdosing the fetus and causing stress to internal organs. Do not ingest, do not use vaginally, do not use rectally. Do not use oils neat, or in high dilutions. This keeps the risk low, and we are looking for low risk and high effectiveness. Low dilutions are still effective. Do not exceed a 2% dilution during pregnancy, ever. Keep the dilution at .5%-1%.

LAST THOUGHTS ON CLINICAL AROMATHERAPY DURING PREGNANCY

Do you have to go the clinical aromatherapy route when pregnant? No, but if you are looking for the safest and most researched methods, it is your best bet. Essential oils may be natural, but they are not to be taken lightly, especially during pregnancy. While there are some things I would do for myself that are not clinically approved, I wouldn't use them on a client, and I would fully inform them of the risks. There are many oils that are classified as pregnancy safe that just don't have the clinical studies to back up those claims. If that is a risk you want to take, just be informed. If you want studies to back up your choices, choose clinical aromatherapy.

Another thing to remember with aromatherapy during pregnancy is that the advice tends to differ from person to person, even in a clinical setting. This can vary by the education a person received, and even the country they are from. You will find different practices in America than in the UK. The important thing to remember is that you know the research behind things and are confident in your knowledge and use of aromatherapy during pregnancy. If you are working with a professional and they are trying to get you to do something that you do not feel comfortable with, do not be afraid to speak up. Only do what you personally trust and know the associated risks of. And still avoid doing things that are labeled as high risk in pregnancy.

ESSENTIAL OILS DURING PREGNANCY (A NON-CLINICAL LOOK)

This section will be a general look at pregnancy; what is considered safe to use but is not backed by clinical studies. It is your choice whether or not you want to follow a clinically based practice for pregnancy but be aware of the risks that are involved. When in doubt, reach out to a professional for help. These are the general recommendations for pregnancy. This content might seem a little repetitive in this section, but for those people who want to skim for the information they need, I feel it is important to repeat certain points with each different route of aromatherapy you could take during pregnancy. Although this is a more detailed look at essential oils in pregnancy from a non-clinical perspective. I do apologize if it seems repetitive in this section, but I needed to get all of the information regarding what using essential oils looks like in pregnancy from both standpoints, and this is how I know how to do it. Since clinical takes a different approach as far as the oils used, some of the advice looks the same although there are more essential oils regarded as safe for use in pregnancy outside the clinical standpoint. I also felt it was important to write this chapter specifically for referencing, as I knew some people would want to reference the clinical portion, or non-clinical portion, of this chapter.

DISCOVERING YOUR PREGNANCY

After discovering you're pregnant, immediately discontinue use of essential oils. Whether your method of use is topical or inhalation, stop using all of them. Absolutely never, ever ingest essential oils during pregnancy, even if you do so in a safe (professional) manner. If you work with an aromatherapist who encourages ingestion during pregnancy, find another aromatherapist. While I discourage use in the first trimester, as many other aromatherapists do, and advise people to wait until their second trimester to utilize essential oils, there are a few things that someone might turn to essential oils for, morning sickness being the main one. Please find alternative methods before using essential oils. Again, do NOT ingest essential oils. If you find that you need them to help curb nausea, then inhalation is your best bet. Ginger or peppermint in your diffuser or in a personal inhaler would be acceptable to use.

Try other methods first. Use essential oils as a last resort! There are many other natural ways to help curb nausea. Ginger in tea, candy, or infused with some honey can really help. Peppermint tea is useful for nausea as well. If you find you need some aromatherapy, consider using a hydrosol instead. A peppermint hydrosol is a much safer option and can be ingested to help with morning sickness (about 1 tablespoon with at least 8 ounces of water). Try those options before attempting to use essential oils, and really stick with not using essential oils the first trimester, unless nothing else is working for you.

SECOND TRIMESTER

Once you enter the second trimester, essential oils use is acceptable. It is believed that some essential oils do cross over to the placenta, so it's important to keep dilutions low and only use pregnancy safe essential oils. Some essential oils that are safe to use during pregnancy (and breastfeeding) are:

- Basil - *Ocimum basilicum ct estragole, Ocimum basilicum ct linalool, Ocimum basilicum ct cinnamate*
- Bergamot - *Citrus bergamia, Citrus aurantium*
- Bergamot, mint - *Mentha aquatica, Mentha citrata*
- Cardamom - *Elatteria cardamomum*
- Cedarwood - *Cedrus atlantica, Cedrus deodora, Juniperus mexicana/ashei/ virginana*
- German and Roman chamomile - *Matricaria chamomilla, Matricaria recutita, Chamomilla recutita, Anthemis nobilis, Chamaemelum nobile*
- Cinnamon leaf - *Cinnamomum verum/zeylanicum*
- Clary sage (for labor, clary sage can potentially kick start labor) - *Salvia sclarea*
- Clove *Eugenia caryophyllata, Syzygium aromaticum, Eugenia aromatica*
- Copaiba - *Copaifera officinalis, Copaifera langsdorfii*
- Cypress - *Cupressus sempervirens*
- Dill - *Anethym graveolens*
- Eucalyptus - *Eucalyptus globulus, Eucalyptus radiata, Eucalyptus dives*
- Fir - *Abies alba, Pseudotsuga menziesii, Abies sibirica*
- Frankincense - *Boswellia carterii/sacra, Bowswellia serrata*
- Geranium - *Pelargonium graveolens*
- Ginger - *Zingiber officinale*
- Grapefruit - *Citrus paradisi*
- Helichrysum - *Helichrysum italicum, Helichrysum stoechas*
- Ho wood (ho leaf linalool) - *Cinnamomum camphora spp glavescens*
- Jasmine - *Jasminum grandiflorum, Jasminum officinale*
- Juniper berry - *Juniperus communis*
- Lavender - *Lavandula angustifolia, Lavandula officinalis, Lavandula vera, Lavandula latifolia, Lavandula spica*
- Lemon - *Citrus limon*
- Lemongrass - *Andropogon flexuosus, Cymbopogon citratus, Andropogon citratus*
- Lime - *Citrus aurantifolia, Citrus x aurantifolia, Citrus x latifolia*
- Mandarin - *Citrus reticulata, Citrus nobilis*

- Marjoram - *Thymus mastichina, Origanum majorana, Origanum hortensis, Origanum hortensis ct carvacrol/ct linalool*
- Neroli - *Citrus x aurantium*
- Orange - *Citrus sinensis, Citrus aurantium var sinensis, Citrus x aurantium*
- Patchouli - *Pogostemon cablin, Pogostemon patchouly*
- Pepper - *Piper nigrum, Schinus molle, Piper nigrum*
- Peppermint - *Mentha piperita*
- Pine - *Pinus sylvestris, Pinus nigra*
- Rose - *Rosa x damascena, Rosa damascena*
- Rosemary - *Rosemarinus officinalis ct camphor/ ct cineole*
- Sandalwood - *Sandalwood spicatum, Santalum cyngornum, Fusanus spicatus, Eucarya spicata, Osyris lanceolata, Santalum album*
- Spearmint - *Mentha spicata*
- Spruce - *Picea mariana, Picea nigra*
- Tangerine - *Citrus reticulata, Citrus nobilis, Citrus tangerine*
- Tansy, blue - *Tanacetum anuum*
- Tea tree - *Melaleuca alternifolia*
- Vetiver - *Vetiveria zizanioides, Andropogon muricatus*
- Ylang ylang - *Cananga odorata, Cananga odorata genuina*

  This is by no means an exhaustive list, but please know which oils are safe and which are unsafe. I only included those I thought were most popular, and only species of them that I thought were most readily available.

  Some companies will list if a product is pregnancy safe, however many do not. They also can't make any kind of claims and will most likely defer you to your care provider rather than saying something is safe. I recommend finding a complete list and keeping that on hand to reference for which essential oils are considered safe or not. Also always ask your care provider before using essential oils.

  What ways can we use essential oils in pregnancy? Inhalation and topical use are the two main ways. As I stated before, do not EVER ingest essential oils during pregnancy. Doing this is extremely dangerous, especially ingesting essential oils that are deemed unsafe for those who are pregnant. Essential oils are extremely potent and ingesting them during pregnancy can cause many problems for you and your baby.

- Inhalation - diffuse essential oils for emotional issues, nausea, headaches, or congestion.
- Topical - apply to sore muscles, aching bellies, and to treat pelvic or skin problems.

Also remember to only use a .5%-1% dilution during pregnancy. As I mentioned before, it is believed that essential oils cross over to the placenta, so it's important to keep dilutions low. If you find that you need a higher dilution for targeted issues, I wouldn't go higher than 2%. It might seem silly to take such precautions, but it's much better to be safe than to have something happen and be sorry.

Limit your essential oil use. I know that in this day and age of easily accessible essential oils, alongside bad advice, people are prone to using them all day long. Please do not do this during pregnancy. In fact... please don't do this ever, but especially while pregnant please be aware of how much you are using essential oils. Limit your use to a few times a day. Have a purpose when you are using them. Do you need emotional support? Relief from muscle aches? Then use essential oils if you want. But don't pop on your diffuser for the heck of it and diffuse all day long. You are more prone to reactions the longer you expose yourself.

SOME WAYS WE CAN USE ESSENTIAL OILS TO SUPPORT A PREGNANCY

Essential oils can be incredibly useful throughout a pregnancy for addressing many complaints, including morning sickness, stretching/itching, painful bellies, joint issues, emotional issues, pain relief, and support through labor. I personally used essential oils in my labor for pain relief, I used them to help with my morning sickness, extreme aches/pains, and to help support me throughout my labor. My favorite oils to use included clary sage (for labor), chamomile, peppermint/spearmint, lavender, dill, and a few others.

There are many great ways to apply essential oils during your pregnancy. Personal inhalers loaded with oils like peppermint, dill, or ginger can help with morning sickness or nausea. An oil rub with those same oils can also help curb sickness. You can help to support labor with essential oils like bergamot, clary sage, geranium, tea tree, lavender, Roman chamomile, jasmine, rose, frankincense, black pepper, orange, and spearmint, either by helping you relax, providing pain relief, or helping to progress labor. I used rose, neroli, peppermint, clary sage, and orange to help calm me down and encourage labor.

You can also use soothing or moisturizing oils like chamomile, geranium, or frankincense to help with those belly itches. Mix them in with a lotion or create your own with some shea butter for a soothing belly balm. Pain relief oils can help with those pregnancy cramps as well. I don't know about you guys, but I got the most wicked leg cramps during my pregnancy!

REACTIONS DURING PREGNANCY

Things get a little weird during pregnancy, so it's entirely likely that you could have a reaction to an essential oil that you have never had any issues with before. If this happens, discontinue use, wash the area thoroughly and gently, and don't go back to that essential oil until after pregnancy. You might want to consider discontinuing the use of essential oils altogether in the event of a reaction, but if other oils are not bothering you, it is fine to continue using them after the reaction has cleared. However, be aware that this could be a lifelong reaction from here on out. I used to be lactose intolerant until after my pregnancies. Things can really change when you get pregnant. Don't let this discourage you! There are many great oils out there, even if you can't use a specific one anymore.

Do not apply more essential oils over a reaction. If you are unsure of the cause, go ahead and stop all usage. Your body is not detoxing if you have a reaction, and you could cause more stress to your pregnancy by continuing to use that essential oil (or any oils) and it's just not worth the risk. It's also important to note that pregnancy is not the time to try new essential oils. If you are just getting into essential oils during your pregnancy, start slowly, but if you have already been using essential oils, use what you have and try to avoid introducing an oil you have never used before. Consider working with a professional if you have never used essential oils before and would like to use them during your pregnancy.

WHAT ABOUT ESSENTIAL OILS IN MY EVERYDAY PRODUCTS?

I also want to touch on this because we often replace things in our daily lives with essential oils. These are typically in our daily face routines, cleaning products, and various other bath/beauty products as well. Many companies also turn to essential oils to scent their products, and we cannot be too sure of their dilutions. I know that many companies use essential oils in their products and never share safety information or how high of a dilution they are using. It is quite popular nowadays for natural-minded brands to utilize essential oils in their products, ranging from skin care to cleaning products. We can gauge what kind of dilutions are used in pre-bought items by seeing how far down the essential oil is on their ingredients list, but that's far from a precise measurement.

Is it unsafe to use these items if they contain essential oils? Honestly you guys, I'm unsure. Especially with a store-bought product. So, my advice would be to make sure any product you are using contains pregnancy safe essential oils. I am less concerned about using products that wash off compared to something like a lotion or a lip balm, however, it is still important to remember that there are not a lot of studies (if any) that have investigated the impact of essential oils on pregnancy. The recommendation is to abstain from essential oil use in the first trimester. Ultimately, do what you are comfortable with, and always discuss with your care provider what is best for you. It does not do any good to be overly stressed out over daily products. Is using a product containing minimal amounts of essential oil going to cause an issue? Most likely not, especially considering we live in a world that is obsessed with synthetic fragrance and very readily okays the use of such products in pregnancy.

So, is something containing essential oils going to be worse for us than spraying ourselves down with fragrance our entire pregnancy? I do not believe so, and I can understand the want/need to find more natural alternatives. The rules of safety do still apply, and there are certain essential oils that need to be avoided in pregnancy. I don't recommend buying or making products with wintergreen (or other unsafe essential oils), still don't recommend ingesting essential oils, and insist that topical maxes for pregnancy should still be adhered to. Also, if you feel most comfortable ditching fragranced items (essential oils or artificial fragrance) then do so. You really can't be TOO safe during pregnancy in my opinion. It truly is better to be a little overcautious. Then again, I would like to say that it does no one any good to be stressed. If swapping your product is easy for you then by all means, swap it. If trying to find alternatives is going to be more work, stress, and too difficult for you then please do not feel like you must swap products out. In the end, when it comes to pre-made products, it is entirely up to you to decide if you want to keep using them or swap them for fragrance free options.

LABOR SUPPORT

This section is pretty straightforward on the subject of how to safely utilize essential oils. The same rules apply, however there are some essential oils that are not baby safe, but which are safe to use during pregnancy. Peppermint, for example, is one I highly recommend not diffusing or using around a newborn baby. In fact, I would encourage women to avoid diffusing anything at all once their baby does come. Newborns are fresh and sensitive and can be easily overwhelmed. Leave that time for bonding with your baby and save the oils for later. Oils are not needed once labor has passed, unless you are using them for healing, and in that case your baby should not be smelling those essential oils.

You can utilize essential oils in a variety of ways to ease your labor. Diffusing to create the atmosphere you desire or picking scents that are calming or stimulating to help relax and encourage labor are great strategies. Using massage oils with your partner to help ease the aches and pains of labor is also worth considering. The possibilities are endless when it comes to using essential oils to aid in labor. I would like to note that if you are planning a water birth, please avoid the topical use of essential oils (or adding oils to the tub) before getting into the water, since there is a chance that you could leave some oil floating in the water and it could react with your baby once you birth them into the pool. If you don't plan to give birth in a pool and are just using it for pain relief, then go ahead and apply topically. However, if there is even the slightest chance of a pool birth, be mindful of this risk. If using topically and getting into the pool, make sure the oil is totally soaked in or gently wipe it off. On that note, do not add essential oils to a birthing pool; opt for a foot soak instead, with a foot spa, and always dilute the oils in a carrier before adding them to the water.

The same rules also apply as when using oils during pregnancy. Respect the topical max and use safe oils for labor. Be mindful to not leave the diffuser running for hours either - stick with 30 minutes on, 1 hour off. Give yourself a break; too much essential oils use can stall out labor and lengthen your birth time. When picking essential oils for birth, there is a list of oils that are great for birth and labor support, but it's also whatever you like. So long as an oil isn't contraindicated for those who are pregnant, then if it helps you go ahead and use it. I personally loved having rose, neroli, and clary sage for my birth. I also used a little mandarin and peppermint as well in my diffuser. Different oils can help at different times during your labor. Let's break them down:

- Basil: Anxiety
- Bergamot: Anxiety, blood pressure, childbirth pain, transition
- Virginian cedarwood: Anxiety
- German chamomile: Back pain during labor
- Roman chamomile: Anxiety, blood pressure
- Clary sage: Blood pressure, childbirth pain, contractions, transition
- Cypress: Anxiety, childbirth pain
- Eucalyptus: Back pain during labor

- Frankincense: Anxiety, childbirth pain
- Geranium: Childbirth pain, contractions
- Ginger: Back pain during labor
- Grapefruit: Transition
- Helichrysum: Blood pressure
- Jasmine: Anxiety, childbirth pain, contractions, transition
- Juniper berry: Back pain during labor
- Lavender: Anxiety, blood pressure, childbirth pain
- Lemon: Anxiety, blood pressure, transition
- Lime: Anxiety, transition
- Mandarin: Transition
- Marjoram: Anxiety, contractions
- Melissa: Anxiety
- Neroli: Anxiety, blood pressure, contractions
- Orange: Anxiety, blood pressure, childbirth pain, transition
- Palmarosa: Anxiety, blood pressure
- Patchouli: Anxiety, transition
- Pepper, black: Back pain during labor, contractions, childbirth pains
- Peppermint: Back pain during labor
- Pine: Back pain during labor
- Rose: Anxiety, blood pressure, childbirth pain, transition
- Rosemary: Back pain during labor, transition
- Sandalwood: Anxiety
- Spearmint: Transition
- Vetiver: Anxiety
- Ylang ylang: Anxiety

Woah! That's a lot, I know. You certainly don't need to utilize this entire list. Use your favorites and let this list be a guide. You do not necessarily have to use these oils for this intended purpose. If one works for you for whatever purpose, then that's awesome! Diffuse oils to help support your emotional health in labor, to help calm you down, and to help get into the mindset to deal with the pain. Use oils topically to help with labor pains, contractions, and any other pains along the way. Again, if you are planning a water birth do not use essential oils and then get into the tub, as this could taint the water and cause a reaction while your baby is being birthed. Wait until the oils are absorbed into your skin, or gently wash them off before getting into the water. Do not add essential oils to your birth tub either!

Also, remember that public spaces like a hospital, or even some birthing centers, might not allow you to diffuse in the room. A personal inhaler of some sort can be super helpful in these situations. Diffusing at home before heading to your birthing place can also be helpful if you are like me and you don't really want to use oils in active labor, and might only use them in early labor. Pre-making topical applications can help as well, like a massage oil for your partner to use on you, or a lotion to help with contractions. There are many ways to use oils that don't necessarily involve diffusing directly. It's important to be mindful of policies, and make sure to ask before diffusing (and definitely ask them before you go into labor as well, you might not remember to ask in the moment!) just to be sure.

CLARY SAGE

There is some debate about the safety of clary sage during pregnancy, as it contains sclareol, which is believed to induce labor. However, objectively looking at clary sage, it looks like the sclareol content is too low to cause this issue. Many women do report that after using it their labor started soon after, or it really helped speed the process along. My general recommendation is to avoid the use of clary sage during pregnancy and save it for labor instead. There are many other great essential oils to use that can help. Until there are more studies done on clary sage and its effects, it is best to avoid using it during pregnancy. If you are wondering if Clary Sage will induce labor though, I have tried inhaling sage twice, and using it topically once, to see if it induces labor and I have had no luck. I don't think anything except Pitocin will kickstart labor unless you are truly ready.

BREASTFEEDING:

A lot of what I have already discussed also applies to breastfeeding, but there is one big difference to consider: your new baby. I recommend not using oils on or around your baby until at least 3 months (although waiting longer is ideal). That means no diffusing, no topical use that would interfere (where they could be exposed to it, smell it, or have it rub off on them) and being aware that essential oils do have a possibility of crossing over in your milk. To avoid this, keep topical applications to .5%-1%. If you do feel you need a higher dilution for targeted issues, there is some grace, and for one time use you could go as high as 5%. But I don't recommend using a 5% dilution often; you should make it a rare occurrence.

Some quick basic guidelines are that children under 1 should use a .2% dilution and children over the age of 15 months can use a .5% dilution. I will be covering essential oil use with children and babies in a later chapter (Ch.10). Refrain from diffusing around your baby. Use a personal inhaler instead or diffuse in another room away from the baby. Do not use topically on your baby until they are over 6 months. Essential oil use should be rare in infants, and you can always use a hydrosol instead of an essential oil. You can begin to introduce diffusing slowly after 3 months, in a large and well-ventilated room. Watch for reactions and stop use if any fussiness/reaction occurs. Again, this is covered in far greater detail in another chapter (Ch.10). My personal recommendation is to wait on the oils, as there is rarely a need for it under the age of 2 anyway.

Avoid applying essential oils to your breast, but if you do choose to, make sure to wash off gently before feeding. A large part of the bonding in breastfeeding is smell, and too much essential oil use can interfere with that. I personally waited 3 months to use essential oils myself, but you do not have to do this if you are keeping them away from your baby.

RESOURCES TO CHECK OUT

If you want some more in-depth information and a deeper look at aromatherapy, check out these other books that I love.

PREGNANCY, BIRTH AND BABY CARE WITH ESSENTIAL OIL, BY REBECCA PARK TOTILO:

This was one of my all-time favorites, with a complete guide to using oils, a list of pregnancy safe oils, and recipes for certain ailments. I used this book the most. However, I would caution you that there is internal use recommended by it, but overall, this is a great book.

WOMEN'S AROMATHERAPY, BY PAM CONRAD:

This is one of the best books to have, especially if you want to learn about the safest and most studied aromatherapy practices for pregnancy. It's easy to read and really explains everything and cites all sources. I recommend this book to anyone wanting to know more about aromatherapy for women in general.

Whether you are looking for some natural remedies or already use essential oils in your life, aromatherapy is a great way to get some help and support during your pregnancy. Knowing how to do so safely is vital, and hopefully this chapter shed some light on just that. It's important to be informed on what appropriate and safe essential oil usage looks like, and how to achieve the desired results. When in doubt, reach out to a professional and make sure you know how to appropriately use oils in pregnancy and are confident in it before proceeding. By knowing the risks, you can make the best-informed decision for you and your family. There is so much to cover when it comes to pregnancy and breastfeeding, but at the end of the day using aromatherapy in these cases is all about being informed, knowing the risks, and following the safety. There are many things that are considered safe in pregnancy that simply lack sufficient studies to prove it. For many, it's just about using what they feel comfortable with and being safe while doing so. Know what's safe and be informed.

CHAPTER 10: ESSENTIAL OILS WITH BABIES AND CHILDREN

Using essential oils with babies and children isn't difficult. However, once again due to the fact that there is so much misinformation out there, it can be difficult to know what is safe or to trust that something is safe. Even when you do find professional help or ask someone who is trained, the advice you'll receive will vary. Some people say we can use essential oils right from birth with babies, while others advise you to wait even longer than the 3 months or 6 months I stipulated earlier. There really aren't a lot of clear guidelines on use with babies and children, but I will share what I learned through all my studies and personal experience. I would like to note that even though there are safety guidelines on using essential oils with babies and children, there really isn't a reason to be using them under the age of 2. Just because you can, does not always mean you should. Babies are sensitive, and rarely have a need for essential oils. So, while I can provide the best information for using essential oils with babies, please take caution and care when doing so.

Before we start on this chapter I do want to note, again, that I do not recommend much use of essential oils (if any at all) on babies. There often isn't a need, and most of the time using the herb or a hydrosol works just as well and is much safer/gentler than an oil. I am only including this chapter so that if someone does choose to use essential oils with a young child, they at least know what is safe. It might seem overly cautious, but with so much bad advice out there, it is so much better to be safe with our little ones.

KNOW WHAT IS SAFE

Many essential oils are unsafe for children, despite being marketed otherwise. Certain blends are often marketed towards babies containing ylang ylang essential oil, which is absolutely not to be used topically on children 2 and under. While safe for diffusing, many recommendations with these blends will have you rubbing the oil (sometimes un-diluted) onto your baby, and even diffusing at all hours of the day/night. Many kid safe lines are anything but safe. Several large companies have "kid safe" lines that are lacking in safety guidelines for children and probably shouldn't be used at all on babies or children, despite them advertising it is safe to do so. Most large market immunity blends are not safe either, since they contain eucalyptus which has cautions for use on children under the age of 10. Yet, somehow these blends are often marketed as totally safe to be used around young children. Once you know what is safe and what isn't, you can begin to use oils confidently with your little ones.

KNOW WHEN TO START

When can you start using essential oils on your baby? I know some people just begin applying and diffusing the minute their baby comes home... but that just isn't safe. My rule of thumb is at least 3 months (diffusing) but preferably 6 months, maybe even longer. Rarely is there a need for essential oils under the age of 2. Also, when I say 3 months, I mean it's okay to use oils around or near your baby but not necessarily ON your baby! You should also exercise caution and the utmost care when diffusing around an infant. This timeframe is really just a go ahead to begin using essential oils on the adults in the household once more. Very rarely is there a topical need for essential oils so young. I will detail how to safely begin using essential oils with children so that if you do choose to do so, you are educated on the safety guidelines before doing so. My recommendation is to wait at least 6 months to use oils with your baby, but there isn't really a need for it when your child is under the age of 2.

Starting with diffusing gently is your best bet. Small increments, in a large, ventilated room, is the way to go. When I started diffusing again after my youngest was born, I let the diffuser go for only 5 minutes. Slowly, we worked to be able to diffuse for 30 minutes at a time. Do not exceed 30 minutes with children, as this can cause reactions or irritations and 30 minutes 3-5 times a day is better than letting the diffuser run for hours anyways. Always start small when diffusing, once a day, and then work up to multiple times a day. Start with one oil at a time, see if there is a reaction, and then slowly move onto other oils. Use less drops in the diffuser as well, with 1-3 drops max for younger ones. Studies on the use of oils with babies are sparse, and I found in my own experience that I was simply diffusing for me or my toddler and not for my baby. I just didn't reach for essential oils to use without a purpose on my baby when she was that young. I instead reached for essential oils for me, while making sure they were still kid safe because I knew my baby would be exposed to them. I personally didn't start topical use until at least over the age of 1, unless there was a need. Waiting until 2 is ideal, but you can safely utilize oils topically at a younger age. Do not use topically under 6 months, at the earliest, as a baby's skin is much thinner, and their immune system isn't very resilient yet.

KNOW YOUR DILUTIONS

Kids are not the same size as adults. That may seem obvious, but the thought that you can use the same amount of oil on a child as an adult is more common than you might think. For ages 2-10 use a 1-2% dilution, and for toddlers if you are looking for daily use I would stick with a .5% dilution. For kids ages 1-2 do not exceed a .5% dilution, and under age 1 a .1% dilution is best. It's important to get dilutions right with children. If you are wanting to use multiple oils in a mix, then mix the oils together before adding the appropriate amount of drops to your carrier. And speaking of carriers - always use a carrier. NEVER use essential oils neat on children or babies. Plant Therapy has a ton of information about dilution, so definitely go check out what they have to say on dilution for kids.

TEST, TEST, TEST

While I don't recommend topical use of essential oils under 6 months (at minimum, but waiting even longer is better), when the time comes it's important to test the essential oils of choice before using. To do this, dilute the oil to the appropriate amount for the age and apply to the inner part of their elbow, then cover with a bandage for 24-48 hours. Check for reactions. If a reaction occurs, discontinue use and gently wash the area in warm water and unscented soap. While tedious, it is important to test each new oil, and this is especially the case with younger children and babies. Oftentimes, reactions take a while to show up in children, so please be aware of this. Many people recommend testing oils neat - do not do this. Dilute to the dilution you plan to use to patch test, and make sure you are using a carrier oil that you know your child isn't allergic to so that your results are not skewed by this possibility.

ALWAYS HAVE A PURPOSE

As much fun as it is to bathe yourself in oil (seriously though, don't do this) we cannot take this approach when it comes to children and babies. Always have a clear purpose in mind when using essential oils. Consider if there is something else that can accomplish what you're looking to accomplish. Instead of using an essential oil for an upset tummy, maybe try a gripe water, a hydrosol, or some natural herbs. Instead of mood lifting oils in babies, try to find other ways to soothe them first. It's better to explore other options before turning to essential oils, especially for young children and babies. Also remember that babies naturally do stuff adults don't and this doesn't mean they need "fixed" with essential oils. Instead of thinking about using essential oils for sleep, consider that new babies aren't even supposed to be sleeping through the night anyway, so they really don't need some calming lavender before bed! Lavender is not an issue but use a hydrosol instead of the essential oil to get that lovely lavender scent. Essential oils are potent and should be a last resort when it comes to babies, which leads me to my next point and alternative option for aromatherapy in young ones.

HYDROSOLS

Especially in babies, a hydrosol is a much better option. They are milder, gentler, and so versatile. Consider using a hydrosol in place of an essential oil. They aren't as commonly known as essential oils, but most companies sell hydrosols alongside essential oils.

What are hydrosols? They are the leftover plant water from the process of distilling to produce essential oils, and they are so much gentler than essential oils as well. They still have many of the same benefits and are safe to use even with newborns. Essential oils shouldn't be used on kids younger than 3 months (and it's even better to wait 6 months or longer), and a hydrosol is a perfectly safe option to use in place of an essential oil.

So, what can we use a hydrosol for, and which hydrosols are on the market? You can find a few hydrosols in health food stores like Whole Foods, but if you want a better selection, online is the way to go, as most essential oil companies sell hydrosols as well. Always buy directly from the manufacturer, and not from a third-party source like Amazon. This guidance applies to both hydrosols and essential oils.

SOME OF MY FAVORITE HYDROSOLS ARE:

- Lavender: I use this for diaper rash, as a bedtime spray, also in a bumps and bruises spray. It can help to alleviate pain, soothe a rash, and calm down a child. Spritz onto pillows, sheets, and even pajamas to help ease into bedtime. Spray right onto the diaper area to provide soothing relief from diaper rashes and spray onto/around bumps and bruises and scrapes to help aid healing and provide relief. It smells wonderful and is perfectly gentle for little ones.
- Tea tree: I use this mainly for diaper rashes and fungal issues, but it can also be a deodorizer. Spray into shoes to help curb the little kids' feet stink! Use as a deodorant in teens/adults. Use for diaper rash/fungal infections.
- Chamomile (Roman): A nice calming/soothing hydrosol, this one is also great to have for skin conditions. Soothe eczema and cradle cap with it. Add some hydrosol to your baby's bottle to help aid with gas and digestion (for ages 6 months+, please seek an aromatherapist for help with dilutions and do not ever give a child straight hydrosol). Use at bedtime with lavender to help ease into sleep and calm down. Alternatively, German chamomile hydrosol is great for sunburn and teething. Just be sure to check those names on the bottle to make sure you have the right hydrosol.
- Geranium: Great for anxiety. This is a wonderful one to have on hand for those hesitant little ones, or even for adults. Spritz around and breathe in to help provide a nice aura of calm for those anxious moments. This is a stimulating one, so not great for bedtimes.
- Rose: Restorative for the skin, though that is not so important for little ones. It just smells great, and I like to use it as a natural perfume that doesn't disturb my little ones. They get a kick out of getting a little spritz of 'perfume' as well, since they love the scent and it's gentle for them.

Whether gas, colic, tantrums, or skin conditions are what you're looking to address, a hydrosol can most likely do the trick. I highly encourage parents to look into getting some of these before turning to essential oils. While oils are great tools, it's much better to pick the gentler route before jumping to the big guns. And hydrosols are much safer for little babies and newborns.

When taking a hydrosol internally, it is important to note that you need to dilute it as well. This makes it easier to take, and kids will probably prefer not to taste it. Having taken some hydrosol internally one time (tea tree hydrosol), it was so gross, and I nearly threw up, this is more for your enjoyment than anything. Adding the hydrosol to some water or to another drink will help make this more palatable especially for children. 1 tablespoon to 8 ounces of drink is a fine dilution.

HERBS

Herbs are another alternative that can be used with children that can help with so many things that people usually try to take care of with essential oils. Instead of rubbing copaiba or clove essential on your baby's gums, consider a clove and catnip teething tincture instead. These are made with whole cloves and low doses of catnip and make for the perfect teething solution for little ones 4 months and over. You can also utilize herb infused oils or balms instead of essential oils for things like diaper rashes or eczema. Calendula is a great skin healing herb that is an option for both of those things since it will really help to heal and soothe any kind of skin irritation.

If you are looking for reputable places to buy herbs or herbal remedies, I recommend checking out Mountain Rose Herbs for bulk herbs and Earthley Wellness for pre-made herbal remedies. Earthley Wellness always lists what age certain products are safe for, and they have many products perfect for under the age of 1.

I would like to note that even though herbs are milder than essential oils, there are still things to be aware of and certain herbs that shouldn't be used with children. I prefer to stick with pre-made items for my family, as it makes it easier for children and babies. It is very important to look up if a particular herb is safe for you and your little one before using it, but luckily there are many resources online that will steer you in the right direction. Please know what you are doing before utilizing herbs or buy from a trusted company that has age labels and safety protocols listed on their products.

MY FAVORITE KID SAFE HERBS FOR HOME USE:

- Chamomile
- Lavender
- Calendula

This little list is pretty much safe for all ages, though I recommend testing out anything new before using it on your baby's skin. You can make some soothing skin balms with these herbs that are so much safer and gentler than essential oils. This is all I will say on herbs, and I strongly encourage everyone to do their own research if they want to use herbs with their family. As this is an aromatherapy book, herbs will simply be a highlight and it's important to know more information before you proceed with using them. I can also only vouch that the herbs I listed are kid safe. Many herbs are, but I know the ones I listed are kid safe.

SHOULD KIDS INGEST ESSENTIAL OILS?

Never. Do not ever allow them to do this. If you are an adult, you may do as you please. While my stance is to discourage casual daily ingestion, or ingestion without guidance, I will always say children should not ingest essential oils. I don't have a lot to say on this; kids just don't need to be ingesting essential oils. It is never safe, never acceptable, and never beneficial. In the event that your child does swallow some essential oil, call poison control and encourage them to drink some milk (full fat milk is best, or if you are breastfeeding, offer the breast as often as possible) or a carrier oil like olive oil, if possible, to help slow the spread of essential oils throughout their system. In most cases, nothing more than monitoring them is necessary, but for more directions poison control is equipped to handle these things.

WHAT IF MY CHILD HAS A REACTION?

Like I mentioned before, if there is a reaction, discontinue use and wash the affected area. However, reactions can look very different in each person. Reactions can even arise from diffusing. Look for weird rashes when introducing new oils and watch for any breathing problems or complaints of headaches. All these things are reactions. Stop using the essential oil altogether if they occur, wash clothing and furniture that might have any residue, and make sure all traces of the oil are washed gently off your child. Avoid reactions by respecting dilutions and diffusing guidelines. Reactions severe enough to necessitate seeing a doctor would be things like extreme respiratory distress, or rashes/allergic reactions that are rapidly spreading or persisting for more than 48 hours.

WHAT ARE SOME OILS TO START WITH CHILDREN?

Beginning to use oils can be a little scary, especially if you don't know which essential oils to start with. So here are some oils that I think are great starting oils (especially for younger kids):

- Frankincense
- Roman chamomile
- Tea tree
- Lavender
- Dill
- Mandarin
- Ho wood
- Spearmint
- Black spruce

Pick one or two from this list (I HIGHLY recommend Roman chamomile and tea tree to start) and test them out. See how they work; these might be the only 2 oils you need for a while. Once your child is over the age of 2, all kid safe oils (make sure they are truly kid safe, and safe for ages 2 and up) are pretty much fair game. I still don't recommend just diving in, even if your child is older, but you don't need to be as cautious when introducing oils if your child is 2+. The younger they are, the slower you should go. I never really used essential oils with any of my children until they reached the age of 2. I would occasionally use essential oils myself, but never topically until they were over the age of 6 months.

COMPANIES THAT OFFER A TRULY KID SAFE ESSENTIAL OIL LINE:

- Plant Therapy
- Eden's Garden
- Simply Earth (they don't have a specific line, but they have the age each oil is safe printed on every bottle)

I have only included companies that I have looked at in depth and trust. While this is intended to be a brandless aromatherapy book, it is also important to share safe information. This means information on what is truly safe for children. I have personally looked over each kid safe line these companies offer and looked at the background information of the companies. I feel confident in recommending this list and you can decide for yourself which of these you feel comfortable using. Each of these companies clearly lists if their oils are for kids and what ages they are safe for. This is not intended to pick out which is better or to make any other company look bad. This is simply me looking at essential oils objectively and comparing the kid safe lines with the facts on what is safe.

To finish off this chapter, I am going to share a list of essential oils that are safe, and what ages they are safe for. Please remain mindful of the fact that this is just from an objective standpoint, and much like essential oils and pregnancy, there are not very many studies showing what is safe with babies and children. Once again, this is going to be a sharing facts kind of thing, intended to present you with the information necessary for you to make the best-informed choice for yourself. I am only going to include the more common essential oils. If something is not listed, you need to look some reputable sources to find out if it is safe. I would also like to add that just because something is considered safe doesn't always mean it is safe for your child. As I have said, the need for essential oils under the age of 2 just isn't present, and I would encourage you to find alternative methods and only turn to essential oils if nothing else has helped. Essential oils are not the only aspect of aromatherapy, they are simply one aromatic therapy, and we can reap these benefits from many other sources such as herbs and hydrosols. It is also important to note that while an essential oil CAN be safe for all ages that does not mean we should be using them on newborns. Wait until at least 3 months (or longer) before using essential oils and wait at least 6 months (or longer) to use essential oils topically on a child. Follow proper dilution guidelines for children and the essential oils as well.

ESSENTIAL OIL AGE GUIDELINES

OILS SAFE FOR ALL AGES (FOR TOPICAL AND INHALATION UNLESS OTHERS LABELED AS ONE OR THE OTHER):

- Amyris – *Amyrsi balsamifera*: No topical max, always dilute before applying to skin
- Angelica – *Angelica archangelica, (Himalayan) Angelica glauca (angelica seed)*
- *Angelica archangelica*: Topical Max is .8%
- Balsam poplar – *Populus balsamifera*: No topical max, always dilute before applying to skin
- Basil, linalool – *Basilicum ct linalool*: 3.3% Max dilution
- Basil, methyl cinnamate – *Basilicum ct methyl cinnamate*: 15% Max dilution
- Basil, estragole – *Basilicum ct Estragole*: .1% Max dilution
- Basil, hairy – *Ocimum americanum*: 30% Max dilution
- Basil, holy – *Ocimum tenuiflorum, Ocimum sanctum*: 1% Max dilution
- Basil, lemon – **INHALATION ONLY** – *Ocimum x citriodorum*
- Basil, Madagascan – *Ocimum gratissimum*: .2% Max dilution
- Basil, pungent – *Ocimum gratissimum*: .8% Max dilution

- Bay, West Indian – *Pimenta racemosa*: .9% Max Dilution
- Benzoin – *Styrax benzoin, Styrax pralleloneurus, Styrax tonkinensis*: 2% Max dilution
- Bergamot – *Citrus bergamia, Citrus aurantium*: .4% Max Dilution
- Bergamot, mint – *Mentha aquatica, Mentha citrata*: No topical max, always dilute before applying to skin
- Carrot seed – *Daucus carota*: No topical max, always dilute before applying to skin
- Cassia – **INHALATION ONLY** – *Cinnamomum cassia, Cinnamomum aromaticum*
- Catnip – *Nepeta cataria*: No topical max, always dilute before applying to skin
- Cedarwood (Atlas, Himalayan, Texas, Virginian) – (Atlas) *Cedrus atlantica*, (Chinese) *Chamaecyparis funebris, Cupressus funebris*, (Himalayan) *Cedrus deodara*, (Port Orford) *Chamaecyparis lawsoniana*, (Texas) *Juniperus ashei, Juniperus mexicana*, (Virginian) *Juniperus virginiana*: No topical max, but always dilute before applying to skin
- Chamomile (German and Roman) – *Matricaria chamomilla, Matricaria recutita, Chamomilla recutita, Anthemis nobilis, Chamaemelum nobile*: No topical max, always dilute before applying to skin
- Cilantro – *Coriandrum sativum*: No topical max, always dilute before applying to skin
- Cinnamon bark – *Cinnamomum verum, Cinnamomum zeylanicum*: .01% Max dilution
- Cinnamon leaf – *Cinnamomum verum, Cinnamomum zeylanicum*: .6% Max dilution
- Cistus – *Cistus ladanifer, Cistus ladaniferus*: No topical max, always dilute before applying to skin
- Citronella – *Cymbopogon winterianus, Cymbopogon nardus*: 18.2% Max dilution
- Clary sage – *Salvia sclarea*: No topical max, always dilute before applying to skin
- Clementine – *Citrus clementina, Citrus reticulata var. clementina*: No topical max, always dilute before applying to skin
- Clove – **INHALATION ONLY** – *Eugenia Caryophyllata, Syzygium aromatic, Eugenia aromatica*
- Coffee – *Coffea arabica*: No topical max, always dilute before applying to skin
- Copaiba – *Copaifera officinalis, Copaifera langsdorffii*: No topical max, always dilute before applying to skin
- Coriander – *Corinadrum sativum*: No topical max, always dilute before applying to skin
- Cumin – *Cuminum cyminum*: .4% Max dilution
- Cypress – *Cupressus sempervirens*: No topical max, always dilute before applying to skin
- Dill – (European) *Anethym graveolens*, (Dill weed) *Anethym graveolens*: No topical max, always dilute before applying to skin
- Peppermint Eucalyptus – *Eucalyptus dives*: No topical max, always dilute before applying to skin
- Fir (all species) – (Douglas) *Pseudotsuga menziesii*, (Silver) *Albies alba*, (Canadian) *Abies balsamea*, (Himalayan) *Abies spectabilis, Abies webbiana*, (Japa

nese) *Abies sachalinensis*, (Siberian) *Abies sibirica*, (Silver) *Abies alba*: No topical max, always dilute before applying to skin
- Fragonia – *Agonis fragrans*: No topical max, always dilute before applying to skin
- Frankincense – *Boswellia carterii/sacra, Boswellia frereana, Bosweillia serrata*: No topical max, always dilute before applying to skin
- Galbanum – *Ferula galbaniflua, Ferual gumbos, ferula erubescens*: No topical max, always dilute before applying to skin
- Garlic – **INHALATION ONLY** – *Allium sativum*
- Geranium – *Pelargonium graveolens, Pelargonium x asperum*: 17.5% Max dilution
- Ginger – *Zingiber officinale*: No topical max, always dilute before applying to skin
- Grapefruit – *Citrus paradisi*: 4% Max dilution
- Helichrysum – *Helichrysum italicum, Helichrysum angustifolium, Helichrysum stoechas*: No topical max (absolute topical max is .5%) always dilute before applying to skin
- Ho leaf, linalool (ho wood) – *Cinnamomum camphora spp galvescens*: No topical max, always dilute before applying to skin
- Hyssop, linalool – *Hyssopus officinalis var decumbens ct linalool*: No topical max, always dilute before applying to skin
- Jasmine – *Jasminum grandiflorum, Jasminum officinale*: .7% Max Dilution
- Juniper berry – *Juniperus communis*:No topical max, always dilute before applying to skin
- Lavandin – *Lavandula x intermedia, Lavandula hybrida, Lavandula hortensis, Lavandin arbialis, Lavandin grosso, Lavandin super*: No topical max, always dilute before applying to skin
- Lavender (Bulgarian, French, Spanish, spike) – (Bulgarian) *Lavandula angustifolia, Lavandula officinalis, Lavandula vera*, (French) *Lavandula angustifolia, Lavandula officinalis, Lavandula vera*, (Spanish) *Lavandula stoechas*, (spike) *Lavandula latifolia, Lavandula spica*: 8% Max dilution
- Lemon – *Citrus limon*: 2% Max dilution
- Lemon balm – **INHALATION ONLY** – (Australian) *Eucalyptus staigeriana*: 3.4% Max dilution
- Lemon eucalyptus – *Eucalyptus citriodora, Corymbia citriodora*: No topical max, always dilute before applying to skin
- Lemongrass – **INHALATION ONLY** – (East Indian) *Andropogon flexuosus, Cymbopogon citratus*
- Lime – *Citrus aurantifolia*, (Key) *Citrus aurantifolia, Citrus x aurantifolia*, (Mexican) *Citrus aurantifolia, Citrus x aurantifolia*, (Persian) *Citrus x latifolia*: .7% Max dilution
- Lime kaffir (combava leaf) – *Citrus hystrix*: No topical max, always dilute before applying to skin
- Mandarin – (including green) *Citrus reticulata, Citrus nobilis*: No topical max, always dilute before applying to skin
- Marjoram, sweet – *Origanum majorana, Origanum hortensis*: No topical max, always dilute before applying to skin

- Marjoram, wild – *Origanum majorana, Origanum hortensis ct carvacrol, Origanum hortensis ct linalool*: 1.2% Max dilution
- Melissa/lemon balm – **INHALATION ONLY** – *Melissa officinalis*
- Myrrh – *Commiphora myrrha, Commiphora molmol*
- Myrtle (honey and lemon) – **INHALATION ONLY** – (honey) *Lealeuca teretifolia*, (lemon) *Backhousia citriodora*
- Neroli – *Citrus x aurantium*: No topical max, always dilute before applying to skin
- Orange blood – *Citrus sinensis*: 1.2% Max dilution
- Orange, sweet (and wild) – *Citrus sinensis, Citrus aurantium var sinensis*: No topical max, always dilute before applying to skin
- Oregano – **INHALATION ONLY** – *Origanum vulgare, Organum unites*
- Palmarosa – *Cymbopogon martinii, Andropogon martini*: 6.5% Max dilution
- Patchouli – *Pogostemon cablin, Pogostemon patchouli*: No topical max, always dilute before applying to skin
- Pepper (all) – (black) *Piper nigrum* (pink) *Schinus molle* (white) *Piper nigrum*: No topical max, always dilute before applying to skin
- Peru balsam – **INHALATION ONLY** – *Myroxylon balsamum, Myroxylon pereirae*: .4% Max dilution
- Petitgrain – *Citrus aurantium*: .4% Max dilution
- Pine (all EXCEPT Huon (*Dacrydium franklinii*) and Ponderosa (*Pinus ponderosa*) - (black) *Pinus nigra*, (dwarf) *Pinus mugo, Pigus montana*, (gray) *Pinus divaricata, Pinus banksiana*: No topical max, always dilute before applying to skin
- Ravensara, bark – *Ravensara aromatica*: .1% Max dilution
- Ravensara, leaf – *Ravensara aromatica*: 1% dilution
- Rosalina – *Melaleuca ericifolia*: No topical max, always dilute before applying to skin
- Rose – *Rosa x damascena, Rosa damascena*: .6% Max dilution
- Rose, absolute – *Rosa x centifolia, Rosa gallica*: 2.5% max dilution
- Rosemary camphor – *Rosmarinus officinalis ct camphor*: 16.5% Max dilution
- Rue – *Ruta Graveolens, Ruta montana*: .15% Max dilution
- Sandalwood (Australian, East Indian, East African, New Caledonian) - (Australian) *Santalum spicatum, Santalum cygnorum, Fusanus spicatus, Eucarya spicata* (East African) *Osyris lanceolata*, (East Indian) *Santalum album*, (New caledonian) *santalum austrocaledonicum*: 2% Max dilution
- Spearmint – *Mentha spicata, Mentha cardiaca, Mentha crispa, Mentha viridis*: 1.7% Max dilution
- Spikenard – *Nardostachys grandiflora*: No topical max, always dilute before applying to skin
- Spruce (all) – (black) *Picea mariana, Picea nigra*, (hemlock) *Tsuga canadensis, Pinus canadensis*, (Norway) *Picea abies*, (red) *Picea rubens*, (white) *Picea glauca, Picea alba*: No topical max, always dilute before applying to skin
- Tangerine – *Citrus reticulata, Citrus nobilis, Citrus tangerine*: No topical max, always dilute before applying to skin
- Tansy blue – *Tanacetum annuum*: No topical max, always dilute before applying to skin
- Tarragon – *Artemisia dracunculus*: .1% Max dilution

- Tea tree – *Melaleuca alternifolia*: 15% Max dilution
- Tea tree Lemon-**INHALING ONLY** – *Leptospermum petersonii, Leptospermum citratum*
- Thyme – *Thymus vulgaris ct carvacrol, cy geraniol, ct linalool, ct thujanol, ct thymol, ct limonene, Thymus serpyllum ct limonene, Thymus zygis ct linalool*: 1.3% Max dilution
- Thyme (Borneol, lemon, serphyllum, spike, zygis) – (Borneol) *Thymus satureioides*, (lemon) *Thymus x citriodorus, Thymus lanuginosus, Thymus serpyllum* (serphyllum) *Thymus serpyllum*, (spike) *Thymbra spicata* (zygis) *Thymus zygis*: 1.3% Max dilution
- Turmeric – (leaf) *Curcuma longa* (rhizome) *Curcuma longa, Curcuma domestica*, (wild) *Curcuma aromatica*: No topical max, always dilute before applying to skin
- Vanilla – *Vanilla planifolia* (bourbon) *Vanilla fragrans, Vanilla tahitensis* (Tahitian): No topical max, always dilute before applying to skin
- Vetiver – *Vetiveria zizanioides, Andropogon muricatus*: No topical max, always dilute before applying to skin
- Yarrow – *Achillea millefolium*: 8.6% Max dilution
- Ylang ylang – **INHALATION ONLY** – *Cananga odorata, Cananga odorata genuina*

OILS SAFE FOR KIDS 2+ (NOT INCLUDING OILS ALREADY LISTED SAFE FOR ALL AGES. FOR TOPICAL USE AND INHALATION.)

- Basil lemon – *Ocimum x citriodorum*: 1.4% Max dilution
- Cassia – *Cinnamomum cassia, Cinnamomum aromaticum*: .05% Max dilution
- Clove – *Eugenia Caryophyllata, Syzygium aromaticum, Eugenia aromatica*: .5% Max dilution
- Garlic – *Allium sativum*: No topical max, always dilute before applying to skin
- Lemon balm – (Australian) *Eucalyptus staigeriana*: 3.4% Max dilution
- Lemon leaf – Citrus limon, *Citrus limonum*: 1.2% Max dilution
- Lemongrass – (East Indian) *Andropogon flexuosus, Cymbopogon citratus*, (West Indian) *Andropogon citratus*: .7% Max dilution
- May chang/litsea – *Litsea Cubeba*: .8% Max dilution
- Melissa/lemon balm – *Melissa officinalis*: .9% Max dilution
- Myrtle (honey and lemon) – (honey) *Melaleuca teretifolia*, (lemon) *Backhousia citriodora*: .7% Max dilution
- Oregano – *Origanum vulgare, Origanum onites*: 1.1% Max dilution
- Peru balsam – *Myroxylon balsamum, Myroxylon pereirae*: .4% Max dilution
- Tea tree, lemon – *Leptospermum petersonii, Leptospermum citratum*: .8% Max dilution
- Ylang ylang – *Cananga odorata, Cananga odorata genuina*: .8% Max dilution

OILS SAFE FOR 6+ (NOT INCLUDING OILS ALREADY LISTED AS SAFE FOR ALL AGES. FOR TOPICAL USE AND INHALATION.)

- Peppermint – *Mentha piperita*: 5.4% Max dilution

OILS SAFE FOR 10+ (NOT INCLUDING OILS ALREADY LISTED AS SAFE FOR ALL AGES. FOR TOPICAL USE AND INHALATION)

- Birch, sweet – *Betula lent*: 2.5% Max dilution
- Cajeput – *Melaleuca cajuputi, Melaleuca leucadendron var cajuputi*: No topical max, always dilute before applying to skin
- Cardamom – *Elettaria cardamomum*, (black) *Amomum subulatum*: No topical max, always dilute before applying to skin
- Eucalyptus Polybractea – *Eucalyptus polybractea ct cryptone:* No topical max, always dilute before applying to skin

Use your own discretion with this list, just because it is listed as safe for all ages or a certain age does not mean that you can go in using essential oils without regarding safety. Always dilute according to age, follow topical maxes, and do not overwhelm your child with essential oils. Less is more.

CHAPTER 11: STORING, GC/MS REPORTS, AND DIY TIPS

Now that we have covered the use of essential oils, including how to use them safely for certain groups as well as what is safe and unsafe for certain groups, let's talk about the rest of what comes along with essential oils.

STORING

Have you ever wondered if you were storing your essential oils correctly, or why your essential oils are smelling a little... funky? Storing essential oils properly is a necessary part of extending their shelf life because doing so avoids oxidation of the oils.

What is oxidation? It's the name of the process when essential oils react with oxygen and their chemical make-up is changed or altered as a result. Basically, they will not hold the same therapeutic benefits they once did, they might not smell the same, or they might even be more irritating to the skin. While all essential oils will go bad like this when stored for a long time, there are some simple steps we can take to stretch the shelf life of our essential oils. Essential oils do not expire in the sense of going bad and spoiling like food does, but avoiding oxidation is still important. While they do not mold, oxidization changes the oil enough that you wouldn't want to use it when oxidized.

Unopened bottles will stay good, as they are not exposed to light or air (when stored correctly away from heat and light) but they do have a shelf life, which is an estimation of how long each oil will last without oxidizing based on the makeup of the essential oil once the bottle is opened. Thinner oils oxidize faster, thicker oils slower. It also depends on how often the bottle is opened, how long it is exposed to the air, and the temperatures it is stored at. Is it away from sunlight and heat? Is it stored in the correct container? Is it tightly sealed? These are all things to consider when storing essential oils.

First things first, what is the shelf life of essential oils? Well, unfortunately. There really isn't a one- size-fits-all answer to this. It really varies with each essential oil, and when it was distilled, bottled, or purchased. It is also important to note that while an essential oil shouldn't oxidize if unopened, this is not always the case, especially if they are stored incorrectly. For some basic guidelines, we can go off this handy little chart:

- Citrus oils have shelf life of 1-2 years
- Plant/floral-based oils have a shelf life of 2-3 years
- Herb/spice-based oils are a shelf lfe of 3-4 years
- Tree/bark-based oils have a shelf life of 4-5 years

However, this is still not really a broadly applicable chart (it's more of a generalization) because some trees have a much lower shelf life, some herbs have a much higher shelf life, and this is further complicated by how the essential oil was distilled. Some distillation methods will affect the shelf life, how it was distilled and collected can affect how long an oil will last before oxidizing. Oils that were distilled and bottled quickly are more likely to have a longer shelf life than ones that didn't have the same care applied to the bottling process. This is why it is important to trust the company you are purchasing from.

It also depends on environmental factors, as mentioned before, and how often it is opened and how it is being stored. Most companies will list the shelf life of each oil they sell, so I recommend looking at that before buying. If a company doesn't have the shelf life reach out and ask, and if they cannot answer I would caution against purchasing from that company. The most important thing is to store the oils correctly and check to make sure they still smell/look/feel alright. If it smells different, looks different, or is suddenly causing a reaction or not acting the same when applied topically, it could be oxidized. Discontinue the use of that oil in cases of oxidization.

Next, make sure the oils are stored in dark glass bottles. If you see essential oils in plastic or clear bottles, do not buy them. Essential oils degrade plastic, and clear bottles let more light in than amber bottles, which can ruin or break down the essential oils. This also brings me onto my next point.

Avoid sunlight and heat. Keep your essential oils stored in a cool, dark place. This can really look different for everyone. Some people keep them out on a shelf, which is fine-if it's not one in direct sunlight or heat. I do not recommend hanging an essential oil shelf in direct sunlight. I keep mine in an essential oil box in my basement, or one of my colder rooms. Some people even go as far as storing their essential oils in a box in the fridge. All of these are great choices, although I don't recommend storing essential oils just in the fridge without another container to isolate them from your food as it might make the food taste funky! Likewise, being in close proximity to food could affect the oils—especially if it's something like garlic or onions. Even in amber bottles, the sun can still break down essential oils. This is true for carrier oils as well, so all essential oils and carrier oils should be stored away from the sun. The sun breaks down a lot. Have you ever left colored paper in the sun? Then you will have seen how one side fades drastically, and long periods in the sun can affect just about anything.

It's important to keep essential oils out of the heat. Since they are volatile plant substances, they are prone to change when exposed to things like air/heat/light. To ensure that they stay good for their entire shelf life, we need to keep them away from these things. I wouldn't store essential oils above 70/72 degrees Fahrenheit, but 65-40 is probably best for essential oils. You also don't want them freezing, so keep them away from freezing temps. In case you were wondering, yes, if it gets cold enough, they can freeze! It will take extreme temps for this to happen and is only a concern if something is being shipped in negative degrees (or if you happen to put your essential oils in the freezer-don't do this). Please note that some essential oils are thicker than others and will require some warmth to get them moving. Roll these oils between your palms in the bottle, or dip into warm (not boiling) water for a few seconds to get them flowing again.

Be sure to cap your essential oils properly after use, and don't leave the cap off as this will expose them to air. The more air that gets into the bottle, the more prone they are to oxidizing. This is also why most essential oil brands have that plastic seal stopper (orifice reducer) in the bottle, as it allows less air to get in. The orifice reducer also helps make it easy to get single drops of essential oil from the bottle. If an essential oil doesn't have this stopper, I wouldn't purchase it. Make sure that those caps are on snugly, allowing for less air to enter. Do not open essential oil bottles (break the seal) until you need them. If you want to open a new bottle of essential oil (maybe you just want to smell it), but you know you won't be using it for a while then reconsider opening it until you need it. A sealed bottle lasts longer, especially when stored correctly. This will lessen air exposure and lengthen shelf life. But look, I get it if you are excited and want to smell your new oil right away! Just keep in mind that if you open the bottle, it will drastically shorten the shelf life.

Another good tip is to buy smaller bottles of essential oils, especially those that are more expensive or have a shorter shelf life. Unless you know that you are going to be using a 30ml (about 1.01 oz) bottle relatively quickly, then it's better to opt for a 10ml or a 5ml. That way you can use the oil more rapidly and won't be left hanging onto a lot of essential oil just for them to oxidize. The bigger the bottle, the more room for air and the higher the chance of it going bad. Consider transferring half empty essential oil bottles to smaller bottles if you aren't using them up that quickly (keeping old 5ml bottles around can be helpful for this, or even sample size essential oil bottles which you can find on Amazon easily).

These storage rules also apply to DIYs and products that you make. Store away from heat/light/air and keep in appropriate containers. I will touch more on this in the DIY section. If you are looking for some good storage containers for your oils, I recommend an essential oil box or fabric pouch. You can find these on Amazon (boxes), or Etsy (fabric pouches and boxes) and they can really help you keep oils organized, as well as away from sunlight.

DIYS

Have you ever seen a DIY, wanted to try it out, but realized the recipe was flawed? Like when it says to add essential oils to water but the oils don't mix in with the water? There are super simple ways to fix DIY mishaps but following essential oil safety and formulation. Too often, I'll see people sharing recipes online without thinking about how to properly formulate them to make them last and work optimally. I can't even remember how many times I have picked up a book and was horrified at the DIY advice it was giving. Even though there are so many recipes online (and in books) that neglect to take safety into account, it doesn't mean we can't use any of them. As long as we know what to look for and what to change/add, we should be able to make just about any DIY work for us in a way that is safe and effective.

So, let's look at common DIY errors and how we can fix them:

1. **NO EMULSIFIER**: This is a big one in liquid projects. People often make a room or body spray without having any way to bind the oils to the water. It doesn't need to be fancy, but there are several ways we can ensure we aren't risking pure oils dropping on us or our furniture. The easiest ways are to use a carrier oil. Mix the essential oils in a carrier first and then add to the water or mix the oils with some aloe vera gel/jelly—the jelly form, not the liquid form, which is available from Plant Therapy—then add that to the water. Using a carrier like oil or aloe is a decent enough fix, but it's not perfect. You will still want to shake lightly before every use. Other methods you can use include using an emulsifier like a natural solubilizer, which you can easily find online by searching the proper name for it online (Caprylyl/Capryl glucoside). This allows the oils to mix into the water, emulsifying it in simple terms. You can also use polysorbate 20, but the solubilizer is a better option if you want to keep things all natural. A couple things to note: witch hazel and alcohol are not great options (as mentioned before), they just don't work as well as people say, and you aren't doing anything by adding those to a product. Using alcohol as a room spray will also make your furniture more flammable, since you need a proof of 95% at least to truly emulsify essential oils! But aerosol air fresheners are also flammable so I'm not sure people actually care about the flammability of fragrances in our homes.

2. **TOO MANY DROPS**: A lot of DIYs contain large amounts of essential oils, and while it might seem great to use more, this is hardly ever necessary. A simple rule of thumb I like to follow is 1-3% for daily use, 5% for short term use, and 10% for one time use. Kids, pregnant women, and the elderly need a much lower dilution; kids 2+ should use .5%-1%, women who are pregnant should use 1%, and adults over 60 should use 1%. So, if you see a recipe calling for a large number of drops, just use less drops and fit the dilution of the DIY for your needs. If you need some help with dilution, check out the dilution charts earlier in this book, Plant Therapy's blog on dilution, or download my dilution charts for free from my website.

3. **INAPPROPRIATE CARRIERS**: Like I mentioned above, when adding essential oils to water, they will not mix. This can be true of a lot of other things, too. Things to avoid as carriers; witch hazel, plain bath salts (you can use bath salts if you dilute them in a carrier oil first), milk, petroleum jelly (and all petroleum based products), pure water (or anything that is primarily water based), aloe vera gel (Plant Therapy's Aloe Jelly is the exception as it has thickeners), and alcohols with too low of a proof. This is especially true when using essential oils on the skin. You always want a proper carrier that will mix with the essential oil and therefore avoid skin irritation. Alcohol could work if it's high enough proof, but it might be irritating to the skin. For topical use, try a lotion, body butter, or carrier oil. For room sprays, make sure to add something else so it's not just oils and water. This ensures the product will work properly and be safe to use. On that note, carriers are strictly for topical use, and it is not advised to use carriers in a diffuser. Use essential oils, extracts, and absolutes ONLY in diffusers.

4. **DIYS STORED INCORRECTLY**: If you see a DIY recommendation to store the finished product in clear glass containers or plastics that are not approved for essential oils, be wary. Essential oils are potent and can erode containers over time. Something

is best for pure oil projects, and projects containing vinegar. If using plastics for your DIYs (again, not with pure essential oils), go for something made of PET plastics, as this will hold up better for essential oils. My rule of thumb is usually to use glass with liquid or oil DIYs, and plastics with lotions, body butters, and balms. If you see someone recommending using any old plastic container or saying to put blends you make in a plastic container, don't just go grabbing something off your kitchen shelf! Make sure you find an appropriate plastic for it. Also, make sure to store DIYs away from sunlight and heat and do not expose constantly to the air. As DIYs contain essential oils, they are also subject to oxidation. We also need to consider all the ingredients in the DIY and make the shelf life of this new product the same as the shortest shelf life of its ingredients. For example, if I use a carrier oil that has a much lower shelf life than everything else, my shelf life needs to match that carrier oil. Always watch for how the DIY project looks and smells as well and throw it out if it smells or looks bad. A preservative can help extend shelf life, especially in water-based DIYs, but it is not necessary. If you don't want a preservative, just store correctly and recognize that the shelf life won't be as long. Without preservatives, water-based products should be stored in the fridge, especially if they are mixed with anything else like a carrier oil.

DIYs can seem intimidating, especially with all the advice floating around, but knowing the basics of how to make, keep, and store them helps make things a little easier. Ensure that you follow appropriate diluting guidelines and store projects correctly, in accordance with how they are made.

GC/MS REPORTS (GAS CHROMATOGRAPHY/MASS SPECTROMETRY)

So, you're looking at a new essential oil company and see they have GC/MS reports. Awesome! But hey... when you click on them, you really can't make heads or tails of what they you're looking at! Trust me, I've been there, and honestly, I am still there sometimes. I'm not sure I am the best person to write about this, but if I am able to understand a report even a little, then anyone can. You don't need to be a scientist to know what to look for, and it isn't too complicated to find the key information necessary to know if the essential oil you want to buy is good. If someone like me can figure out (kind of) what I am looking at, then anyone can figure this out.

I will insert a sample of a (fake) GC/MS report below for reference but remember that each company will have a different looking report. They should still contain what the essential oil is made up of, who signed off on the report, and if they contain anything else besides pure essential oil.

Company Name

GC/MS Batch NO. 12345

Essential Oil: Clove

Botanical Name: Syzygium aromaticum

Country of Origin: Indonesia

Key constituents in this batch of clove	%
Eugenol	80%
eugenol acetate	10%
β-caryophyllene	9%
alpha Humulene	1%

Comments from X inspector: comment comment comment

Company name and address

Make sure you have the report that corresponds with the correct batch. If you want to purchase clove oil, make sure the report you are reading says clove. If you are having issues with this, customer service should be able to help in most cases/companies. Unfortunately, a lot of the time you won't be able to get the specific batch number until you purchase the oil, but companies should still offer the reports online which should include current and past reports (usually stretching back at least 2 years).

First, look for the essential oil name—Latin name—and the country of origin. If any of these are missing, it's a red flag and honestly, I wouldn't purchase them. This tells us exactly what essential oil this is and is helpful to know which type is being used for safety issues.

Second, look for any adulterants. While you could look at each individual constituent, you would probably then have to google each one, or you could scroll down to the bottom and see the conclusion of the report to see if it has any adulterants. This is usually in the form of a comment or chart from the inspector. This is the simplest way, and it's super easy to do. Most companies are not going to sell an oil that contains adulterants, but if one does, make sure you know how much of the oil is contaminated and whether you are comfortable purchasing. Absolutes will always have some contaminants, as they are not true and pure essential oils, so this might be an example of a report having contamination. There should not be anything in the essential oils except for the chemical constituents known to be in that particular oil (besides the solvent from absolutes) and this includes not being diluted with a carrier oil unless specifically sold as a diluted option.

Next, look up what the essential oil is made of. You don't need to be an expert to know this, but it does help to be aware of the main components of certain oils. For example, the cardamom from Plant Therapy has a main component of 1,8 cineole BUT their cardamom contains less 1,8 cineole than other brands. Does this mean it's a fake? I reached out to Plant Therapy and found out that due to where this cardamom is grown, it contains about 5% less 1,8 cineole than other cardamoms. Plant Therapy is known for having batch specific oils, so while cardamom is usually unsafe under the age of 10 (due to the high 1.8 cineole content) Plant Therapy's version is safe for ages 2+. You would have to consider if this is something you feel comfortable purchasing and using, but judging by the fact that they are open in the reports and transparent when asked, I have no doubt that this is the real deal. It just might not be as effective as other cardamoms that do contain a higher 1,8 cineole content. Each essential oil contains a range in which each chemical constituent is present in the oil, and this range is what consider normal for that essential oil. For example, English lavender typical contains 20-35% linalool. If there is more or less of this constituent, something might be off about this oil.

Basically, as a result of looking at the chemical components of certain essential oils, we can see if they match up to what they're supposed to be. This isn't really something that we have to know or even do, but it does help when looking at essential oils. Especially those that are marketed kid safe. High 1,8 cineole oils are not kid safe, so if an oil is marketed as kid safe and contains above 35% 1,8 cineole, it is not safe for kids. It's just something to be aware of. I am certainly not an expert in the chemical composition of essential oils, and I really wish I was able to just list them off the top of my head, so you know what to look for, but being aware and just knowing the percentage that oils contain is a great start. What we are really looking for here is transparency with these reports, and if you have questions then customer service should be able to help. At the very least, they shouldn't just shut you down and should be willing to provide the information. If you do have any questions about the chemical components in an essential oil (like if they are safe for kids or not), feel free to reach out to me and I can help you to the best of my ability.

Lastly, we should look and see that this report was looked at and signed off on by an analyst. You do not have to know them personally but googling them might not be a bad idea. Basically, if you can't find anything at all about this person, I would maybe think it was forged.

That is all I really look for in my GC/MS reports. While they do include the test results, I am not a scientist, so I don't really understand them. But I feel that I don't have to understand the actual report portion, so long as the company is honest and open about their results. So, I look for these main things to make sure it's pure, has the information needed to ID the essential oil, and is able to tell me what chemical components make up the oil. I just do this so that I am familiar with what to look for and so I know what a report should be. Once you are sure of all these things, you are good to go. You do not have to understand the entire report to be able to tell if the essential oil is pure, and in the normal range it should be.

To be quite honest here, I do not look at these reports that often if I already trust a company. With a new company, I am more likely to look. But I do not believe that reports should be withheld simply because someone might not understand. We can pinpoint the information we need to know without needing to have a degree. Reports should be readily available, and not just provided after someone purchases. Companies who don't provide them are not companies I would purchase from. It is important to have access to reports, even before purchasing, and if a company tries to hide their reports it is a major red flag to me.

CHAPTER 12: ESSENTIAL OILS AND THEIR CONSIDERATIONS

In this chapter, we will be going over essential oils that have contraindications or interactions with medicines/medical conditions. It is important to know if an essential oil interferes with a medication you are taking. It is important to know if an essential oil could possibly exasperate a medical condition. This is the case for several essential oils. While some are not very serious, some are very serious. Either way, these are things that everyone needs to know and be aware of. I will provide a list of essential oils and the notes that go along with them. It is not a scary list, more so a list of need-to-know information.

MEDICINE/MEDICAL INTERACTIONS:

- Anise *Pimpinella anisum/Illicium verum*: Potentially a blood thinner. Do not use this with blood thinning medications (even aspirin), bleeding disorders, and before/after surgery. This oil is a reproductive hormone modulator. Do not use this if you have endometriosis or estrogen dependent cancers.
- Arborvitae (western red cedar) *Thuja plicata*: Potentially a convulsant - do not use if you have epilepsy.
- Balsam poplar *Populus balsamifera*: Do not use in any form if using drugs metabolized by CYP2D6.
- Basil (estragole chemotype) *Ocimum basilicum ct estragole*: Potentially a blood thinner. Do not use with blood thinning medications (even aspirin), bleeding disorders, and before/after surgery.
- Basil (holy) *Ocimum tenuiflorum, Ocimum sanctum*: Potentially a blood thinner. Do not use with blood thinning medications (even aspirin), bleeding disorders, and before/after surgery.
- Basil (lemon) *Ocimum x citriodorum*: Do not ingest if using diabetes medications or drugs metabolized by CYP2B6.
- Basil (Madagascan and pungent) *Ocimum gratissimum, Ocimum viride*: Potentially a blood thinner. Do not use with blood thinning medications (even aspirin), bleeding disorders, and before/after surgery. Pungent type: Do not ingest if using pethidine, MAOIs, and SSRIs.
- Bay (West Indian) *Pimenta racemosa var racemosa, Pimenta acris*: Potentially a blood thinner. Do not use with blood thinning medications (even aspirin), bleeding disorders, and before/after surgery. Do not ingest if using pethidine, MAOIs, or SSRIs.
- Birch (sweet) *Betula lenta*: Potentially a blood thinner. Do not use this with blood thinning medications (even aspirin), bleeding disorders, and before/after surgery. Avoid salicylate sensitivity or ADD/ADHD. Do not ingest with GERD.
- Black seed *Nigella sativa*: Do not ingest if using diabetes medications.

- Buchu *Agathosma betulina, Baromsa betulina, Agathosma crenulata, Barosma crenulata*: Potential convulsant, do not use with epilepsy.
- Cassia *Cinnomomum cassia, Cinnomomum aromaticum*: Potentially a blood thinner. Do not use with blood thinning medication (even aspirin), bleeding disorders, and before/after surgery. Do not use this internally with diabetes medication.
- Chamomile, German *Matricaria chamomilla, Matricaria recutita, Chamomilla recutita*: Avoid all methods if using drugs metabolized by CYP2D6. Avoid using internally if using drugs metabolized by CYP1A2, CYP2C9 or CYP3A4
- Chaste tree *Vitex agnus castus*: This is a hormone modulator. Do not use if you are getting progesterone therapy, have endometriosis, or estrogen dependent cancers. Do not ingest if you are using hormone replacement therapy, oral contraceptives, or drugs metabolized by CYP2D6.
- Cinnamon, bark *Cinnomomum verum, Cinnamomum zeylanicum*: Potentially a blood thinner. Do not use with blood thinning medication (even aspirin), bleeding disorders, and before/after surgery. Do not use internally with diabetes medication.
- Cinnamon, leaf *Cinnomomum verum, Cinnamomum zeylanicum*: Potentially a blood thinner. Do not use with blood thinning medications (even aspirin), bleeding disorders, and before/after surgery. Do not use internally with diabetes medication.
- Citronella *Cymbopogon winterianus, Cymbopogon nardus*: Do not use internally if using drugs metabolized by CYP2B6
- Clove *Eugenia caryophyllata, Syzygium aromaticum, Eugenia aromaticum*: Potentially a blood thinner. Do not use with blood thinning medications (even aspirin), bleeding disorders, and before/after surgery. Do not use internally if using pethidine, MAOIs, or SSRIs.
- Cypress (blue) *Callitris intratropica*: Do not ingest if using drugs metabolized by CYP2D6.
- Eucalyptus (Macarthurrii) *Eucalyptus macarthurii*: Do not ingest if experiencing cholestasis.
- Fennel (sweet and bitter) *Foeniculum vulgare*: Potentially a blood thinner. Do not use with blood thinning medications (even aspirin), bleeding disorders, and before/after surgery. This oil is a reproductive hormone modulator, do not use with endometriosis or estrogen dependent cancers.
- Garlic *Allium sativum*: Potentially a blood thinner. Do not use with blood thinning medications (even aspirin), bleeding disorders, and before/after surgery.
- Geranium *Pelargonium graveolens, Pelargonium x asperum*: Do not use internally if using drugs metabolized by CYP2B6.
- Ho leaf (camphor) *Cinnamomum camphor ct camphor*: Potentially a convulsant, do not use with epilepsy, do not ingest if using diabetes medications or drugs metabolized by CYP2E1.
- Hyssop (pinocamphone) *Hyssopus officinalis ct pinocamphone*: Potentially a convulsant, do not use with epilepsy.
- Jasmine (Sambac) *Jasminum sambac*: Do not ingest if using drugs metabolized by CYP2D6.
- Lavandin *Lavandula x intermedia, Lavandula hybrida*: Potentially a blood thinner. Do not use with blood thinning medications (even aspirin), bleeding

disorders, and before/after surgery.
- Lavender (Spanish) *Lavandula stoechas*: Potentially a convulsant, don't use this if you have epilepsy.
- Lemon balm (Australian) *Eucalyptus staigeriana*: Do not ingest if using drugs metabolized by CYP2B6.
- Lemon leaf *Citrus lemon, Citrus limonum*: Do not ingest if using diabetes medications or drugs metabolized by CYP2B6.
- Lemongrass *Cymbopogon flexuosus, Andropogon flexuosus* (East Indian); *Cymbopogon citratus, Andropogon citratus* (West Indian): Do not use in any way if using drugs metabolized by CYP2B6. Do not use internally if using diabetes drugs or if pregnant.
- Marjoram (wild) *Origanum hortensis ct carvacrol*: Potentially a blood thinner. Do not use this with blood thinning medications (even aspirin), bleeding disorders, and before/after surgery. Do not ingest if using diabetes medications (Carvacrol chemotype specifically)
- May chang *Litsea cube, Litsea citrate, Laurus cubeba*: Do not use if using drugs metabolized by CYP2B6. Do not ingest if using diabetes medications.
- Melissa *Melissa officinalis*: Do not use internally if using diabetes medication or drugs metabolized by CYP2B6.
- Mugwort (and Mugwort, great) *Artemisia vulgarisms ct camphor/thujone, Artemisia vulgarisms ct chyrsanthenyl acetate, Artemisia arborescens*: Potentially a convulsant (mugwort), do not use with epilepsy. Do not use if using drugs metabolized by CYP2D6 (mugwort, great) and do not ingest if using drugs metabolized by CYP1A2 and CYP3A4 (mugwort, great).
- Myrtle *Myrtus communis*: Do not use if using diabetes medications.
- Myrtle (honey, lemon) *Melalueca teretifolia, Backhousia citriodora*: Do not use if using drugs metabolized by CYP2B6, do not ingest if taking diabetes medications.
- Oregano *Origanum vulgare, Origanum onites*: Potentially a blood thinner. Do not use with blood thinning medications (even aspirin), bleeding disorders, and before/after surgery. Do not use internally if using diabetes medication.
- Palmarosa *Cymbopogon martinii, Adropogon martinii*: Do not ingest if using drugs metabolized by CYP2B6.
- Parsley (leaf and seed): *Petroselinum crispy, Petroselinum sativum*: Do not ingest if using pethidine, MAOIs, or SSRIs.
- Patchouli *Pogostemon cablin, Pogostemon patchouly*: Potentially a blood thinner. Do not use with blood thinning medications (even aspirin), bleeding disorders, and before/after surgery. Do not use internally if using diabetes medication.
- Peppermint *Mentha piperita*: Do not use if you have G6PD deficiency or cardiac fibrillation. Do not use internally if you have cholestasis or GERD.
- Ravensara (bark) *Ravensara aromatica, Ravensara anisata*: Potentially a blood thinner. Do not use with blood thinning medications (even aspirin), bleeding disorders, and before/after surgery. Do not ingest if using pethidine, MAOIs, or SSRIs.

- Sage (Spanish) *Salvia lavandulifolia, Salvia hispanorum*: Potentially a convulsant, don't use this with epilepsy.
- Sage (wild mountain) *Hemizygia petiolata*: Do not ingest if using drugs metabolized by CYP2D6.
- Sandalwood (Australian) *Santalum spicatum, Santalum cyngnorum, Fusanus spicatus, Eucarya spicata*: Do not use internally with drugs metabolized by CYP2D6.
- Tansy, blue *Tanacetum anuum*: Do not use if using drugs metabolized by CYP2D6. Do not use internally if using drugs metabolized by CYP1A2 or CYP3A4.
- Tarragon *Aremisia dracunculus*: Potentially a blood thinner. Do not use with blood thinning medications (even aspirin), bleeding disorders, and before/after surgery. Do not ever ingest this essential oil.
- Tea tree (lemon) *Leptospermum petersonii, Leptospermum citratum*: Do not use if using drugs metabolized by CYP2B6, do not ingest if using diabetes medications.
- Thyme *Thymus vulgaris ct carcarol, thymol, and limonene*: Potentially a blood thinner. Do not use this with blood thinning medications (even aspirin), bleeding disorders, and before/after surgery. Gernaniol chemotype - do not ingest if using drugs metabolized by CYP2B6.
- Thyme (Borneol, spike, zygis) *Thymus satureioides, Thymbra spicata, Thymus zygis*: Potentially a blood thinner. Do not use this with blood thinning medications (even aspirin), bleeding disorders, and before/after surgery. Spike - do not ingest if using diabetes medications.
- Turmeric *Cucuma longa, Curcuma domestica*: Do not ingest if using diabetes medications.
- Wintergreen *Gaultheria procumbens, Gaultheria fragrantissima*: Potentially a blood thinner. Do not use with blood thinning medication (even aspirin), bleeding disorders, and before/after surgery. Do not use internally if you have GERD.
- Yarrow *Achillea millefolium*: Do not use if using drugs metabolized by CYP2D6, do not ingest if using drugs metabolized by CYP1A2 CYP3A4.

If you have any of these conditions or are taking any of the above medications, it is recommended to avoid the use of the oils listed so you can avoid adverse reactions. So, make sure to be thorough and see which essential oils you might have to avoid, or not use in certain ways, depending on the medications that you are on or certain conditions you may have.

PHOTOTOXIC ESSENTIAL OILS:

- Angelica root *Angelica archangelica*: Phototoxic if used over the topical max of .8%
- Bergamot *Citrus bergamia, Citrus aurantium*: Phototoxic if used over the topical max of .4% (cold pressed varieties; there are non-phototoxic varieties also available on the market)
- Cumin *Cuminum cyminum*: Phototoxic if used above the topical max of .4%
- Grapefruit *Citrus paradisi:* Phototoxic if used above the topical max of 4% (cold pressed varieties)

- Lemon *Citrus limon*: Phototoxic if used above the topical max of 2% (cold pressed varieties)
- Lime *Citrus aurantifolia, Citrus x aurantifolia, Citrus x latifolia*: Phototoxic if used above the topical max of .7% (cold pressed varieties)
- Bitter orange/blood orange *Citrus x aurantium, Citrus aurantium subsp amara/ turs sinensis*: Phototoxic if used above the topical max of 1.2% (cold pressed varieties)
- Rue *Ruta graveolens, Ruta montana*: Phototoxic if used above the topical max of .15%

It is important to note that with phototoxic essential oils (phototoxic means having a reaction to UV rays) if you follow topical dilutions, you should be fine. However, it is still recommended that phototoxic essential oils be applied at least 12 hours before any UV exposure (sun, tanning, uv lights, etc.) so take care and caution with phototoxic essential oils.

OILS WITH OTHER WARNINGS/CONTRAINDICATIONS:

- Allspice *Pimenta officinalis*: Potentially carcinogenic
- Anise/anise star *Pimpinella anisum/Illicium verum:* Potentially carcinogenic
- Arborvitae *Thuja plicata*: Noted as neurotoxic
- Basil (estragole) *Ocimum basilicum ct estragole*: Potentially carcinogenic
- Basil (Madagascan and pungent) *Ocimum gratissimum*: Potentially carcinogenic
- Birch (sweet) *Betula lenta*: Noted as toxic
- Buchu (Diosphenol and Pulegone) *Agathosma betulina, Agathsom crenulata*: Noted as hepatotoxic
- Camphor (brown/yellow) *Cinnamomum camphora*: Potentially carcinogenic, brown was noted to never be used
- Himalayan Cedarwood *Cedrus deodora*: Moderately toxic
- Dill seed (Indian) *Anethum sowa*: Noted as hepatotoxic and nephrotoxic
- Fennel (bitter and sweet) *Foeniculum vulgare*: Potentially carcinogenic
- Ho leaf (camphor) *Cinnamomum camphora ct camphor*: May be neurotoxic
- Hyssop hyssopus officinalis ct pinocamphine: Noted as neurotoxic and may be carcinogenic
- Laurel leaf *Laurus nobilis*: Potentially carcinogenic
- Lavender (spike) *Lavandula latifolia, Lavandula spica*: May be neurotoxic
- Lemon balm (Australian) *Eucalyptus staigeriana*: Noted as teratogenic
- Lemon leaf *Citrus limon, Citrus limonum*: Noted as teratogenic
- Mace *Myristica fragrans, Myristica officinalis*: Potentially carcinogenic, and may be psychotropic
- Mugwort *Artemisia vulgaris ct camphor/thujone, Artemisia vulgaris ct chrysanthemum acetate, Artemisia arborescens*: Noted as neurotoxic
- Mustard *Brassica nigra Brassica juncea:* Noted as toxic and noted as do not use
- Myrtle *Myrtus communis*: Potentially carcinogenic
- Nutmeg *Myristica fragrans, Myristica officinalis, Myristica moschata, Myristica aromatica, Myristica amboinensis*: Potentially psychotropic, potentially carcinogenic

- Palo santo *Bursera graveolens*: Noted as hepatotoxic
- Parsley leaf *Cymbopogon martinii, Andropogon martinii*: Noted as toxic
- Parsley seed *Cymbopogon martinii, Adnropogon martinii*: Noted as hepatotoxic and nephrotoxic
- Pennyroyal *Hedeoma pulegioides, Mentha pulegium, Micromeria fruticosa*: Noted as hepatotoxic and nephrotoxic
- Pine (ponderosa and huon) *Pinus ponderosa, Dacrydium franklinii/Lagarostrobos franklinii*: Potentially carcinogenic, noted as do not use
- Ravensara (bark/leaf) *Ravensara aromatica*: Potentially carcinogenic
- Rosemary (camphor) *Rosmarinus officinalis ct camphor*: May be neurotoxic
- Sage (dalmatian) *Salvia officinalis*: Noted as neurotoxic and potentially a convulsant, noted as do not use
- Sugandha *Cinnamomum ceiciododaphne, Cinnamomum glaucescens*: Noted as carcinogenic and noted as do not use
- Tansy *Tanacetum vulgare, Chrysanthemum tanacetum*: Noted as neurotoxic and potentially carcinogenic. Noted as do not use
- Tarragon *Artemisia dracunculus*: Potentially carcinogenic
- Tea tree (Black) *Melaleuca bracteata*: Noted as carcinogenic and noted as do not use
- Wintergreen *Gaultheria procumbens, Gaultheria fragrantissima*: Noted as toxic

It is important to note that these are just possible effects, and usually only likely to happen with overuse of the essential oil or if you ignore the corresponding topical maxes. This list is not meant to scare anyone, and besides the ones that are noted as do not use, most healthy adults can continue to use these oils in moderation and heavily diluted. If you have any kind of medical issue, or are taking medications, then maybe go ahead and skip the oils on the list. However, I feel it is important to note the considerations along with certain essential oils so that anyone who is choosing to use them is fully informed and knows how to go about utilizing them safely. You also will probably not find a lot of these oils on the list, especially ones listed as "do not use" because most companies will not sell an oil that is dangerous. The oils that you can continue to use in moderation (ones like nutmeg and wintergreen) are sold and should have the appropriate safety alongside them when being sold. As always talk to your care provider before using the oils on this list, and also contact a professional aromatherapist if needed.

CHAPTER 13: RECIPES FOR THE WHOLE FAMILY

To end this book, I am going to share some of my favorite recipes which are family friendly and can be adapted to fit the unique needs of yours.

SIMPLE BALM
2 oz carrier oil of choice (almond oil, grapeseed oil, FCO etc.)
2 oz grated beeswax (pellets might make it too hard, but if you have pellets weigh out 2 oz)
Essential oils of choice (use a 1-2% dilution for daily balms and a 3-5% for targeted balms)

Melt the beeswax into the carrier oil over a double broiler. Remove from heat and allow to cool for 2-5 minutes. Don't let the edges harden. Add the essential oils to the desired dilution and mix in well. Add to the desired container and place in the fridge to harden.

HEALING BALM
Dried calendula flowers 2 tbsp
Dried lavender flowers 2 tbsp
¼ cup almond oil
¼ cup shea butter
2 tbsp beeswax
2 tbsp Aztec Clay
5 drops of lavender or tea tree essential oil (optional)

Combine the almond oil and dried flowers and allow the flowers to steep on low over a double broiler for 30 minutes. Be careful not to make the stovetop too hot. Strain out the flowers and add the oil back into the double broiler with the shea butter and beeswax. Melt down the beeswax and shea butter to combine. Once melted, remove from heat and allow to cool for a couple minutes. Add essential oils, if you are using them, and then add in the clay, whisking well to combine. Add to your desired container and set in the fridge to harden.

Use balm for healing, dry skin, eczema, diaper rash, or rashes. Cloth diaper safe.

HOMEMADE LOTION BASE
2 tbsp beeswax
½ cup almond oil
2 tbsp vitamin E oil
2 tbsp cocoa butter
¾ cup water
Essential oils of choice

Heat the almond oil, vitamin E oil, beeswax, and cocoa butter over low heat on a double broiler until melted. Take off the heat and let cool for 3-5 minutes. Using a blender or emulsion blender, SLOWLY add the oil to the water and blend. An emulsion process should start, and the lotion should begin to thicken and form. Continue to add slowly and blend until everything is well combined and a lotion has resulted. It should be slightly thick, but with a nice fluffy consistency that spreads easily.

This will not be as thick as body butter. PLEASE NOTE that since this is a water-based recipe this will need to be stored in the fridge, or you will need to add some kind of preservative to the water before making it into lotion.

If adding essential oils, you can add into the cooled oil and make the lotion as normal, or you can add it into the lotion base and mix thoroughly. This would be the same as buying a lotion base and adding essential oils to it.

HOMEMADE CHAPSTICK BASE
2 tbsp beeswax
2 tbsp shea butter
¼ cup oil of choice (almond, jojoba, or grapeseed is a good choice)
Essential oils of choice

Heat the beeswax, shea butter, and carrier oil over low heat in a double boiler until melted. For a firmer consistency use more beeswax. Remove from heat, allow to cool for a couple of minutes, and then add essential oils of choice. I recommend a .5-1% dilution for Chapstick and that you ensure the essential oils you are using are not phototoxic. Transfer into the desired container and allow to cool. You can check the consistency of the Chapstick by stirring a spatula through the oils and then allowing the spatula to chill in the freezer for a few minutes to harden.

HOMEMADE BODY BUTTER BASE
2 oz shea butter
.5 oz coconut oil
.25 oz grapeseed or almond oil
.25 oz beeswax

This recipe is in oz because this is my main body butter recipe, and I must weigh it out. You will need a scale for this one, because if I convert anything I will ruin this recipe!

Heat the shea butter, coconut oil, grapeseed oil, and beeswax on low over a double boiler until melted. Remove from heat and allow to cool for a few minutes. Add in your desired essential oils and then place in the fridge to cool completely. This will be about 20-30 minutes, or until it has started becoming solid but still pliable and soft. Then take a hand mixer or emulsion blender and start to whip/blend. This might take several rounds of back and forth-whipping, putting it in the fridge, and then whipping again. Continue to whip until it reaches a lovely airy texture and will slide on the skin like butter.

Body butters are a lot thicker than lotions and will leave more of a greasy feeling on the skin than a lotion. These are best used at nighttime. Body butters help to retain the moisture in the skin and are best for extremely dry skin types. I like to use a body butter after a shower or bath.

HERBAL OIL
Herb of choice
For trauma oil use St. John's wort, calendula, and arnica
For skin healing use lavender, Roman chamomile, and calendula
Oil of choice (FCO, olive oil, or apricot would work)

Add herbs to a mason jar, about half to ¾ full. Cover the contents of the jar with the oil, completely soaking the herbs. You might have to shake the jar to fully cover the herbs and add more oil as needed. Place some parchment paper over the jar before adding the lid and then set in a place away from the sun for 4-6 weeks to steep. Rotate the jar daily.

If you want a quicker way to make an herbal oil, you can do 1 cup oil to 4 tbsp of herbs and heat on low for 30-60 minutes in a double broiler. Do not boil. Keep the heat low.

Dried herbs work best for this, but if you want to use fresh make sure to lay them out to dry enough to get all the water out. Especially after washing herbs. Any extra water in this will make the oil rancid. Use an herbal oil by itself or use in any of the recipes for added benefits. Herbal oils are great for children and babies as well.

If you are using multiple herbs, infuse each herb separately in their own jar and then mix the oil in the correct portions when done. Herbal oils are great for using as a carrier oil for topical use of essential oils.

CONGESTION BLEND FOR KIDS
Eucalyptus dives
Spearmint
Black spruce

UPLIFTING BLEND
Lemon
Grapefruit
Mandarin

UPSET TUMMY BLEND
Dill weed
Roman chamomile
Spearmint

BUMPS AND BOO BOOS BLEND
Helichrysum
Frankincense
Lavender

FOCUS BLEND
Spearmint
Basil
Rosemary CT camphor

CALM DOWN BLEND
Roman chamomile
Mandarin
Tangerine

SLEEPY TIME BLEND
Ho wood
Black spruce
Vetiver

FINAL THOUGHTS

Thank you so much for your support and for reading my book! It truly means so much to me to have this support, and to be able to do something to give back to my community. Even if you didn't need this book because you already knew a little about essential oils, I hope you found it helpful in some way. I loved writing this book, and a lot of hard work went into doing so. More work went into this book as I moved towards releasing and eventually officially publishing it. Heck, this whole epilogue might even change by the time I get to that point! But for now, I have FINISHED my book, and I am so stinking excited! This is a project that has been in the works for the last couple years, and that I have been writing/editing for the past year. It really is a huge step forward for me and I am super excited to be able to share my knowledge and make essential oil education affordable and accessible. Again, thank you so much. I hope that you found this book helpful.

RESOURCES

I spent years learning about aromatherapy and essential oils. This means I have found other aromatherapists and sources that I love and incorporate in my daily practice. I recommend picking up any of these books if you want to learn more about aromatherapy and continue past a beginner's level of knowledge. These books are wonderful tools to grow your practice and learn even more.

- Aroma Hut Institute   (for aromatherapy certification)
- NAHA (National Association of Holistic Aromatherapy) website for continuing education and aromatherapy certification guidelines https://naha.org/
- Essential Oil Safety by Robert Tisserand and Rodney Young (for healthcare providers)
- Women's Health Aromatherapy by Pam Conrad
- Aromatherapy and Women's Mental Health by Pam Conrad
- Pregnancy Birth and Baby Care with Essential oil by Rebecca Park Totilo
- Therapeutic Blending with Essential Oil by Rebecca Park Totilo
- The Complete Book of Essential Oils and Aromatherapy by Valerie Ann Worwood
- Hydrosols the Next Aromatherapy by Suzanne Catty
- Aromatherapeutic Blending Essential Oils in Synergy by Jennifer Peace Rhind
- Robert Tisserand, the Tisserand Institute, and the website/blog https://tisserandinstitute.org/

WANT TO CONTINUE LEARNING?

If you liked this book and want to continue getting essential oil tips and education, check out my social media and website. I share daily tips as well as safety information on my Instagram, Facebook, and blog. Follow them here:

- Facebook: Holisticary Aromatherapy
  - Instagram: aromatherapist_tris
- Website: holisticaryaromatherapy.com

GLOSSARY

- Anticoagulant: Inhibits blood clotting
- Aromatherapy: The use of aromatic plant extracts and essential oils in massage or baths
- Carcinogenic: Having the potential to cause cancer
- Chemotype: A chemotype is a chemically distinct entity in a plant or microorganism, with differences in the composition of the secondary metabolites.
- Constituent: Being a part of a whole, a part of what makes up essential oils
- Convulsant: Producing sudden and involuntary muscle contractions
- Distill/Distillation: Extract the essential meaning or most important aspects of
- Essential Oils: Plant extracts that take the most concentrated part of the plant
- Emulsion: A fine dispersion of minute droplets of one liquid in another in which is not soluble (mixable)
- Hepatotoxic: Damaging or destructive to liver cells
- Nephrotoxic: Damaging or destructive to the kidneys
- Neurotoxic: Poisonous to the nervous system
- Phototoxic: Becoming toxic after a reaction to light
- Psychotropic: Relating to or denoting drugs that affect a person's mental state
- Teratogenic: Relating to or causing developmental malformations

www.ingramcontent.com/pod-product-compliance
Lightning Source LLC
Chambersburg PA
CBHW070643030426
42337CB00020B/4139